Hot Mess
—— to ——
Mindful Mom

Hot Mess
to
Mindful Mom

40 Ways to Find Balance and Joy in Your Every Day

Ali Katz

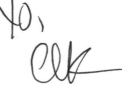

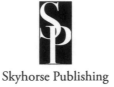
Skyhorse Publishing

Skyhorse Publishing books may be purchased in bulk at special discounts for sales promotion, corporate gifts, fund-raising, or educational purposes. Special editions can also be created to specifications. For details, contact the Special Sales Department, Skyhorse Publishing, 307 West 36th Street, 11th Floor, New York, NY 10018 or info@skyhorsepublishing.com.

Skyhorse® and Skyhorse Publishing® are registered trademarks of Skyhorse Publishing, Inc.®, a Delaware corporation.

Visit our website at www.skyhorsepublishing.com.

10 9 8 7 6 5 4 3 2 1

Library of Congress Cataloging-in-Publication Data is available on file.

Cover design by Jane Sheppard

Print ISBN: 978-1-5107-2106-7
Ebook ISBN: 978-1-5107-2108-1

Printed in the United States of America

This book is dedicated to:

Mark,

I can't imagine my life without your love and unending support.
You have my heart from now until forever.

Adam and Dylan,

Being your mom is truly the best gift I could ever ask for.
You make me proud every single day.

Contents

Introduction

As a mom, do you ever feel that you are just making it through the day until bedtime? If so, I understand. Until a few years ago, I had days like that too, but I realized there was another way—one where I didn't feel that I was simply going through the motions, but instead was savoring every moment of raising my kids. I love my kids with all my heart, and, for them, I wanted to find a way to be not only a better mom, but also a better person.

This book is for moms who want to live a more balanced and mindful life so they can stress less and enjoy more. Our kids grow up so fast. The days turn into months quickly, and if we aren't paying attention, we'll miss them. Focusing on the present moment allows us to soak up all the joy of life and feel fulfilled and happy.

As a certified meditation teacher, self-care coach, and mom of two young boys, I have personally implemented every one of these strategies and techniques into my own life. From the bottom of my heart, these tips changed my life and helped me transform from a Hot Mess to a Mindful Mom.

Some of the topics you will learn more about are:

- Self-care and self-love
- Creating rituals
- Forgiving yourself and others
- Cultivating gratitude
- Mindful eating
- One-minute meditations
- Expanding time

I now feel that I live a life full of meaning. I can appreciate special moments as they are happening, and can see the lessons and growth in the more challenging ones. I have achieved a greater sense of balance between being a mom and being *me*.

Rha Goddess coined one of my favorite quotes, "People will take real over perfect any day." I couldn't agree more. I get extremely real and tell it like it is in this book. I uncover my challenges and struggles, and how I overcame them. I am NOT perfect, and I don't pretend to be, but I have found an easier way—a better way—to be the kind of mom and person that I can feel great about.

I break down my tips into three categories:

- Non-negotiables: things I do every day
- Add-ons: things I do as needed
- Attitude adjustments: personal changes I've made along the way that helped me to grow as a person

These forty bite-sized lessons make it easy to grab an idea and implement it into your life immediately.

Be the mom that is so together everyone else wants to know your secret. Don't wait to make these changes. See every day as a gift, not a chore. You owe it to yourself and your family to find the balance, joy, and happiness in every day. As Shubhanshu Tiwari says, "You cannot change everything around you, but you can create a better world within yourself." You have the power to create an inner landscape of peace and calm that not only makes you feel grounded and secure, but also allows your whole family to benefit as well.

The following forty ideas I share literally transformed my life, and they can do the same for you. Commit to creating your best life right now, and get started!

SECTION 1

Everyday Practices

I'm a wife and a mom. I drive the carpool. I cook (or at least try) even though half the time my family won't actually eat what I make. In theory, I exercise six days a week, but in reality, it's three. I try to spend time with friends, but that doesn't always work out, either. In the midst of this crazy life, I'm also building a business as a meditation teacher and self-care coach. But no matter what, every single day, I still manage to find ways to be mindful.

I like calling myself "everyday spiritual" because I incorporate spirituality and mindfulness into everything I do every day so that even the most mundane tasks have meaning and help me to grow as a person. I am constantly learning lessons, working on forgiving myself and others, and practicing self-awareness. Sure, some days are better than others, but with a deeply ingrained spiritual mindset and a sense of humor, even my off days can feel like a true gift. We can all agree that being a mom is pretty incredible, but it's also really hard. We need tools to help us navigate situations where we don't have all the answers.

Spirituality is an expansive term everyone must define in their own personal way. This is what being spiritual means to me:

- Understanding my connection to the Universe
- Honoring myself as a human being and as part of my family
- Giving and receiving love freely
- Living free from judgment of myself and others
- Creating opportunities to connect with my true self
- Valuing what each individual brings to this world
- Believing that there are forces in the Universe working to help me reach my full potential

You may or may not know what spirituality means to you, and by no means should that stop you from reading this book. My goal is to share the tools that I use to bring spirituality and mindfulness into my everyday life with the hope that they inspire you in some way. I truly feel that these techniques have made me a better person and a better mom. I get pretty personal throughout this book because, mom to mom, you deserve my brutal honesty. Many of the experiences I share may resonate with you, and I encourage you to make a few small shifts—even one change can bring more fulfillment, joy, and meaning to your life.

1

Self-Care

"Self-care is not about self-indulgence, it's about self-preservation."
—AUDRE LORDE

My husband and I bought our house thirteen years ago, when we were engaged. A friend told us about an open house in the area where we were looking, and the description in the paper sounded amazing, so of course we went.

The previous owners had very different taste than we did. The outside was what I lovingly called terra-cotta, but my family called "salmon spread" behind my back. The decor was very Texan, with stars on the doorknobs and an unfortunate amount of duck-patterned fabrics. Even though we knew we had some work to do, we didn't care. Those were just cosmetics. The house would get painted, the bathrooms eventually redone, and the kitchen updated.

Those things aside, the spirit of the house spoke to us. We walked in and immediately fell in love with it. I looked at my then-fiancé and said the magic words: "We have to raise our children here."

We soon found out that the house was listed at the wrong price in the paper—by a lot. Total bummer. We tried to negotiate with the owners, but they wouldn't come down enough, and since there was only so far we could stretch our budget, we had no choice but to walk away and keep house hunting.

Three weeks later we got a call that the owners had changed their minds and agreed to our price, and we got the house. We were beyond ecstatic and jumped on it immediately.

We definitely made a good call. It was a little more space than we needed at the time, but we have grown into the space beautifully, and are raising two boys who play soccer up and down the long front hall daily. I never thought I would appreciate a hallway so much!

Every year, we choose one improvement project for our house. We typically spend all year saving, planning, and prioritizing. Over the years, we have made this house our home. We take care of it and it takes care of us. We put love and energy into the house, and it provides a safe and comfortable space to make wonderful memories as a family and with our loved ones and friends. I can't imagine moving, and don't think we will for a long, long time.

These big improvement projects are exciting, but it is the day-to-day care of my house that allows it to continue to serve our needs and be a nurturing environment for my family. A house requires constant care and attention to maintain. Taking out the trash, changing lightbulbs, dusting, vacuuming, scrubbing bathrooms . . . the list goes on. These chores are non-negotiables unless I want my home to turn into an unkempt mess, especially with two boys running around, but over the years they've become habits.

The more I care for my home, the more of a haven it becomes for myself and my family. Just as I care for my family's home with

love, I care for my own personal, physical home—my body—the same way.

My physical body houses my soul. It is my personal shrine to my spirit. My body carries out loving acts and deserves to be cared for as well. Taking care of my physical and emotional needs is one way that I tell myself that the essence of me is important. I practice self-care as away to honor everything about myself. To be happy and feel complete I require a combination of time with loved ones, time teaching and serving the world, and time to care for myself. It took me a while to figure this out, and these components are weighted differently each day. Sometimes I need more of one than the other, and I do my best to honor my feelings as they arise each day.

I have always been pretty rigid in relation to my calendar and to-do list, and, for a few years, I was downright neurotic. If something was on the list for Tuesday, it would get done on Tuesday come hell or high water. I couldn't go to sleep until every single thing was crossed off my list or I would start to go into panic mode. It took years of living this way to finally realize that nothing terrible was going to happen if I had to be a little flexible—in fact, quite the opposite. As I began to chill out with all the meditation I was doing, becoming less reactive and more responsive, I started to see the bigger picture; the world wouldn't end because of an uncrossed task on my list.

Flexibility trickled into other areas of my life as I started my teaching and coaching business as well. Occasionally a task had to wait, and exercise got pushed off to accommodate my clients' schedules, but I went with it. This time of growth could have been miserable if I wasn't willing to be flexible, but it was exciting and fun instead. I somehow rearranged, and found pockets of time for myself as well as my growing business. I am now trying to cultivate more flexibility in my children because I realize what a gift it is.

I spent years thinking that I was only a good wife and mother if I put everyone else's needs above my own. I thought that martyrdom somehow proved my love. I now realize that by filling up my own cup first, I have so much more to give those that I love; when I feel depleted, my entire family suffers right along with me. As the mom of two young boys, I pretty much must plan my life around their schedule, but I've also learned to incorporate what I need and am willing to do what it takes to make that happen. It could mean waking up at 5 o'clock in the morning to get a meditation and workout in before they go to school if I have a busy work day. It could mean bringing a magazine to flip through at baseball practice if I need to zone out, or scheduling alternating workout times with my husband on the weekends. Sometimes it takes major effort to fit all the pieces of the puzzle together, but it can be done. With practice, I have found ways to meet my own needs without skimping on those of my family.

To me, self-care is synonymous with the word "balance." We need to be productive as much as we need downtime. We must always give to others without forgetting about ourselves in the process.

The most precious commodity we have is *time*. We can't buy more of it, so we better make the most of what we have. Caring for ourselves should be a top priority—caring for ourselves is a vital component of caring for others. I like to think that I am setting a good example for my children. I want nothing more than for them to be happy, healthy, and well-adjusted individuals. In order to do so, they must eat right, exercise, enjoy a hobby, spend time with friends, and learn to appreciate being alone. I can't expect this to come naturally to them, so I feel that modeling healthy behavior is the best thing that I can do as their mother.

The wonderful thing is that there are no rules about how one should care for themselves; it is incredibly personal. For me, meditation is a must—for others, a morning workout might be the most important thing. Maybe it's a healthy breakfast, a weekly manicure, or buying some new workout gear. It could be time at the end of a long day to read, take a hot bath, or indulge in a favorite show. Some people treasure time spent connecting with friends, and others just want to be quiet and not say a word. I talk about many self-care rituals throughout this book, but I'd like to highlight a few here in order to get your brain moving in this direction.

Cultivate "Me" Time

I have a few favorite ways that I nurture and care for myself, and meditation—a *medi*, if you will—is at the top of the list. I like to say that a medi is the new pedi. I love a mani/pedi just as much as the next gal, but if I had to choose one thing to do with any extra downtime these days, it would be to meditate.

If I told you that there would be a present waiting for you every morning if you got out of bed ten or fifteen minutes earlier, would you do it? I would! I love presents, and I think that most people would set their alarm and eagerly hop out of bed without hitting snooze. That is exactly how I feel about my alone time in the morning. It is a gift that I give to myself every day. That time spent in solitude creates a reservoir of calm and peace for me to use throughout my entire day. No matter what my schedule holds, I am committed to waking up early to have this time. Without it, my day doesn't have the same soothing flow and rhythm. I realize that not everyone needs as much time as I do. For some, five minutes of quiet does the trick.

I have a dear friend who sits for five minutes every morning mindfully drinking a cup of hot water with lemon. She feels the warmth of the mug in her hands and follows the sensation of the liquid entering her body. This is her time, and it is what fuels her before her demanding day begins.

My In/Out Rule for Eating

I aim to have healthy eating habits most of the time. What works for me is eating very healthy at home, and indulging a bit more when I am out. At home, I tend to eat only natural sugar, small amounts of mostly goat milk dairy, and healthy carbs. Dark chocolate (72% cacao or higher) is my treat of choice, and I break a square off a large bar once (maybe twice) a day.

I don't have iron-clad willpower outside my home, but I don't feel guilty for treating myself to richer foods when I partake in them. That is why the in/out rule works for me. We mainly eat at home during the week, and I find balance in eating whatever I want, within reason, on the weekends. I am mainly drawn to healthy foods in general, and, as a pescetarian, I am somewhat more limited, but desserts can sometimes get me. I just can't pass up a bite . . . or three.

My Makeup Routine

My love for skincare products and makeup came later in life. I don't know if it was the 80s or growing up in the North, but I didn't wear much makeup when I was younger. I didn't have a knack for applying it, and I had incredible skin back then. I think it was age and sleepless nights as a new mom that that sent me begging for under-eye concealer at the nearest makeup counter.

I started to notice that other moms looked less tired and more pulled together. They weren't caked in makeup, but they looked polished. I began to invest in a few lessons and decent products and

they did make me feel like I looked a bit more awake. My skills improved and makeup became another way to express and care for myself. I still tend to wear natural colors, but it's fun to change them with the seasons. Even on the days that my hair is thrown in a ponytail, you can rest assured that my under-eye circles are covered. I don't do this for anyone but myself. My husband thinks I look beautiful without any makeup, but putting a little extra effort into my appearance makes me feel good. I may live in workout clothes and leggings, but with a little blush and lip gloss I can go from yoga to teaching, to my computer, to driving the carpool. It just works for me.

Special Dates Are a Priority

My husband and I need dates to reconnect and be alone. Even though we talk many times a day, it's different to be at a quiet dinner together. I plan coffee dates with friends because texting doesn't always suffice. Never to be forgotten are dates with my kiddos; at least once a month I try to take each one to do something special. I may soak them up playing gin and sipping hot chocolate at Starbucks or enjoying an ice cream cone together. It doesn't really matter what we do as long as they know that they have my undivided attention without anyone else around.

My husband and I also have a ritual that has helped us as a couple tremendously. It's always fun to be social, so on Saturday nights we often make plans with another couple or two. I don't know if this happens to you, but when groups of couples go out, the men often sit at one end of the table and talk, and the women at the other. As fun as the night is, I usually can't say two words to my husband until we get back in the car to go home! Now, when we have plans with other people, whenever possible we go an hour early and sit at the bar and enjoy a drink and talk. This way, we have a bit of alone time and a real conversation before we meet up with friends.

I treasure the time I spend with loved ones, but the older I get, the more time I need alone, and this is very important to my self-care. I love to read outside in my backyard, take leisurely walks alone or with my dogs, indulge in mandala coloring, or do online Kundalini yoga videos. I set aside time each week to do these things just like any other important meeting on my calendar so that I don't get too caught up in my list of tasks to take time for myself.

Exercise

Exercise is another way that I care for myself, but only by doing things I enjoy. I used to train with a wonderful group of women two or three days a week in the early mornings, and the camaraderie coupled with the workout was incredibly motivating. I hardly even noticed that I was lifting weights, which was something I had never enjoyed in the past.

That group disbanded when our trainer moved, but my motivation and commitment to my body was solidified with that experience. I find as many ways as I can for exercise to be something I enjoy by doing yoga and running outside, which is my absolute favorite activity. It's all about finding what works in my schedule and doesn't feel like torture. I have also started making exercise a social activity, and when someone asks me to grab a coffee, I usually suggest a walk instead. If I can exercise and chat with a friend it is a win/win!

Self-care isn't something that we fit in when we can. It needs to be a priority in our lives, because when we take care of ourselves, we can do a much better job caring for those we love.

2

Self-Love

"Beauty begins the moment you decide to be yourself."
—COCO CHANEL

Who are we without our roles? We often label ourselves as a spouse or partner, a parent, a child, a sibling, a friend, or an employee. I was at a class recently taught by my amazing teacher and mentor Sarah McLean, and we were asked to introduce ourselves to the person sitting next to us. Pretty typical stuff. I heard words buzz around me like the ones described above. We were then instructed to introduce ourselves again using adjectives that were our "soul qualities." Words could be heard floating around the room, such as grateful, open, present, creative, and thoughtful. What if we felt confident enough to introduce ourselves like that all the time? "Hi, I'm Ali. I am enthusiastic, committed, loving, and sincere." It would be so interesting to meet new people and really get to know them on a different level. I want to go to *that* cocktail party or high school reunion!

As much as self-care is about balance, self-love is about acceptance.

It doesn't come naturally to adults to honor and accept our true selves. Our internal ego voice, the one that makes us feel judged and insecure, tends to tell us that we aren't good enough, smart enough, or thin enough. Telling the ego to take a hike is the first step toward practicing self-love. When my ego makes an unexpected appearance, I silently say to myself, "Ego, you aren't invited into my day. Goodbye." I know it sounds kind of silly, but it works. Say it often enough, and when you hear those nasty thoughts creeping in you can create an internal shift to help carry you to a new normal—one where you spend each day being kind to yourself.

How would it feel to get texts from a friend saying things like, "You are such an idiot! Why did you say that?" or "OMG, what were you thinking? That outfit does NOT look good. Who do you think you are?" or maybe even, "You ate that whole piece of cake? You are such a cow!"

I would not be able to delete that person from my contacts fast enough. But the friend that texts sweet messages like, "You are awesome!" or "Even though it didn't work out, you totally gave it your best shot," or even "Don't worry about not getting invited to the dinner, you need time to relax and binge watch *Parenthood* anyway"—I am in love with that friend!

Seventy percent of our internal dialogue is negative, and for some, it is even higher. Start to pay attention.

Here's the thing: we should be our own best friend and biggest cheerleader. Instead, we are usually our worst critic. We all need to be kinder, more compassionate, and less judgmental to ourselves. This is actually one of the essentials of meditation that I teach—*be kind to yourself.*

We are so quick to pass judgment and blame ourselves, but we have a hard time expressing what we actually like about ourselves.

Why can't we celebrate our successes? When someone I care about does something great, I want to know about it. I want to honor and celebrate them, and that goes for their kids too, if they have them.

Parents bond so easily by discussing their children's issues and challenges, but the moment you say something good about your kid, you are obnoxious. Why is that? Why do we feel so much more comfortable commiserating about negative influences? Where are the celebrations?

One morning I came downstairs and my son, who was eight at the time, surprised me and had everything ready for school. He felt so grown up and capable. He made breakfast for himself and his brother, he packed their snacks, and he even decorated his brother's lunch bag. He got their toothbrushes ready, laid out their backpacks, and lined up their shoes. The only thing missing was my tea (which we can work on for next time).

I was so incredibly proud of him. It was one of those moments as a parent where you glimpse your child as an organized and mature individual and you know that they will somehow get it together to take care of themselves eventually. His initiative was something I wanted to celebrate, so I uploaded pictures of his handiwork to Facebook. I honestly didn't care if others thought I was bragging. That's their problem, not mine. I began writing a new story that day. Now when my kids do something great, I may ask a friend, "Can I celebrate something with you?" I set the tone that I want to share something special, not that I am going to brag about my kid. I have reframed it in my mind, and I encourage others to do the same by modeling that it is okay to share the good stuff too.

I am also on a one-woman mission to teach people how to accept compliments with grace and ease. Think about how many times someone gives you a compliment and you come back with a reason why it isn't true. Someone may say, "I love your top," and you reply, "This is so old." A much better response would be, "Thank you." Someone may say, "You look pretty today." Instead of, "I hardly slept a wink last night and the bags under my eyes have bags," how about "Thank you," instead? Learn how to accept a compliment. Honestly, the person saying something nice is not only trying to make you feel good, but they feel good when they share a sweet sentiment. Don't take that away from them! Just say "Thank you," even if you don't believe what they said. Just say it and smile. I challenge you to start giving more compliments as well. See how good it feels, and then notice how others react. It is pretty amazing.

Here's the deal—we shouldn't measure our self-worth and value based on outside praise. Love is first and foremost an inside job. We can practice self-love by celebrating all of the wonderful things about ourselves.

The more abundantly we love ourselves, the more our lives change for the better. Love becomes our default setting.

Try this . . .

Take a moment and make a list of all the wonderful things about yourself that make you feel proud and confident. I bet there are a ton when you really start thinking. You can throw the list away when you are done if you like, so go crazy and don't hold back. What comes to mind? Are you funny, kind, beautiful, sexy, thoughtful, or wild? Are you a hard worker, generous, and unafraid to take risks? Celebrate yourself and all of your amazing qualities. There isn't another YOU in the entire Universe. You are a gift to this world. You are perfectly YOU.

Be generous with yourself; give yourself the benefit of the doubt and learn to not take everything so seriously. We all say things we regret, and wish we could have a "do-over" at times. I used to drive myself crazy replaying conversations in my head and imagining that

I had offended someone or made them upset, when in reality that was never the case. I would usually call to offer an apology after staying awake all night worrying, only for the person to tell me that they had no idea what I was talking about. We build these events up in our heads when we really just need to move on and let them go.

I am not suggesting that we don't filter. Of course, we should always try to be on our best behavior, but we aren't perfect. When we say or do something that we regret, we need to learn, grow, and then release the guilt.

Believe me, this all takes practice. It takes a lot of retraining to overcome years of beating ourselves up, but the commitment to self-love is worth it. You have the rest of your life to reap the benefits of this work. It feels amazing to have a positive perspective on life.

Don't be nervous about bringing up self-love to your kids. If you notice that they are beating themselves up with unkind words, talk to them about what kind of story they can tell themselves instead. If you help your kids reframe situations in their mind, they begin to do it on their own. It just takes practice. We can also help them by modeling self-love for them. When you make a mistake, try not to use negative words about yourself, even though it can be hard. It is easy for something like "I am such an idiot" to fly out of our mouths when we make a mistake. Begin to be mindful of the language you use around your kids. Being on our best behavior for them is great practice!

As adults, nobody can help us with self-love. It is an inside job which we must accomplish as part of living a balanced and happy life. The first step is awareness. Simply notice what words you use in your thoughts about yourself. Catch yourself in the act of negative thinking and reframe those thoughts to be more positive and loving. With time, new, healthier habits will form.

3

Meditation—the Daily Vitamin for Your Soul

"Meditation, because some questions can't be answered by Google."
—UNKNOWN

One of my favorite things about meditation is that there is something for everyone. There are as many reasons to meditate as there are people meditating. Many people come to meditation for very practical reasons, such as:

- Reducing stress
- Lowering blood pressure
- Becoming less reactive and more responsive
- Boosting the immune system and decreasing allergies
- Regulating sleep and digestive patterns
- Increasing productivity and creativity
- Reducing chronic pain and migraines

- Increasing neuroplasticity (literally changing your brain)
- Increasing memory and ability to focus
- Increasing feelings of gratitude and compassion
- Improving presence
- Improving problem solving and decision-making

I, on the other hand, came to meditation from a very spiritual place and more to connect with the world around me. I don't often tell the whole story, but since I promised brutal honesty, here goes . . .

I like to say that the Universe hit me over the head with spirituality.

About five years ago, I went to a seminar at my synagogue. Truthfully, I only went because a dear friend of mine was in charge of the event and I would have felt bad not showing up. Before the guest speaker began talking, my friend leaned over and told me that the speaker's sister was a famous spiritual medium. I had never thought about mediums before, but it sounded interesting. By the end of the evening, I was happy that I dragged myself out of the house.

Two weeks later, I was in Los Angeles visiting some friends. One of them mentioned at dinner that she recently had a reading with a medium who was amazing. Well, wouldn't you know, it was the same person that I had heard about at my temple. Kind of a fun coincidence, right?

A week later, I was randomly watching a show that someone had recommended to me, and a small part of the storyline involved a medium—it was getting kinda crazy now. That same week another friend told me that her mom recently had a reading with an amazing medium . . . yes, the same one. Definitely crazy now!

I promptly decided that there have definitely been many signs throughout my life that I have missed, but this one couldn't be denied. I had to have a reading with this medium; without a doubt, the Universe was pointing me in that direction. Whether you believe in what spiritual mediums do or not, there is no denying the amazing synchronicities in this story. It was like flaming arrows were pointing me to her.

I had to wait six months for my appointment, so, in the meantime, I began reading this woman's books. She seemed extremely gifted, and I was counting down the days until our conversation.

Most people come to mediums to connect with a specific loved one, but that wasn't my situation. I had absolutely no idea what to expect; I was simply open-minded and excited—and, in the end, I was absolutely stunned by her accuracy and insight. I don't want to get too deep into a conversation about guardian angels and spirit guides because I understand that these ideas don't resonate with everyone. However, I connected with loved ones in profound ways, and it brought immense joy and peace to my life. I will share just one example of her accuracy for all the skeptics out there: she knew what I had been talking about in the car with my kids that very morning.

The reading changed my life in many ways. I instantly felt more connected to the world around me, as well as loved and supported beyond measure. I wanted to continue to communicate with my guides and loved ones. In the books I had read, and on my call, this medium suggested meditation. I had no clue that this simple self-help practice would change my entire life.

I had never thought about meditation before, but decided to give it a try. I bought a book on the topic, read a few pages, and went for it. Even though I had no real clue what I was doing, when I sat in stillness it felt really natural and just plain good. So I kept going.

I had overcome many ups and downs in my life but never actually acknowledged any of the stress that accompanied these experiences. Denying my feelings and pasting a smile on my face were my self-preservation tactics of choice. I had no connection to my intuition, very little self-awareness, and I often felt like I was floundering on the inside. People who know me may be surprised to hear me describe myself who way, but that was what was behind the brave face.

After about six weeks of daily eight-minute meditations, I began to notice unexpected changes happening. For years I had lived with a ball of anxiety lodged in the center of my chest. I don't know where it came from, but I've felt it for as long as I can remember. During that sixth week, I was walking my dog and I stopped dead in my tracks. All of a sudden I realized that the fiery ball that I was convinced was going to one day explode in my chest was gone. I fluctuated between thinking, "Where did it go?" and "Who freaking cares?" I felt so free. As I walked home I realized that I had no clue how this happened, but the only thing that had changed in my life was that I was meditating.

The instructional book I read didn't go into a lot of detail about the benefits of meditation, so I hadn't been anticipating anything like the mental, physical, and emotional transformation that occurred over the next few months and years. With more consistent practice, I began to:

- Feel more present, calm, and grounded
- Have more patience
- Wean myself off caffeine because I felt so great after my morning meditations I didn't crave it anymore
- Feel more gratitude and compassion
- Feel more connected to my intuition and sense of self

- Tackle my sleep issues and get myself off of Ambien (after being addicted for more than two years)
- Slow down and truly enjoy special moments
- Gain confidence in myself and my abilities
- Increase my stamina
- Place less emphasis on material things
- Prioritize the relationships that deserved the most time and energy
- Feel less reactive

I could go on and on, but you get the gist. Before I began meditating, on the outside my life looked the way I had always wanted it to. I had an amazing husband, two wonderful kids, a beautiful home, and financial security, but inside I was reeling. I was always making choices I regretted and never felt secure in myself. I truly felt that meditation was the catalyst to an amazing metamorphosis. I then knew with 100 percent certainty that a very big part of my life's purpose was to teach and inspire others to bring meditation into their own lives as well.

Looking back, it's crazy to think that those snippets of conversation about a spiritual medium got me to where I am now. The Universe definitely had a plan for me!

As a meditation teacher and self-care coach, I strongly suggest that all my students start their day with meditation. I always tell them that I am not the "meditation police," so if first thing in the morning doesn't work for them we can figure out another game plan, but meditating first thing is great because you start your day from a calm, peaceful, and grounded place. It also prevents meditation from becoming one more task on your to-do list.

My practice started with an eight-minute meditation each morning. I stuck with that program for eight weeks, and as I began to feel more confident in my practice I began to slowly add time to each session. For the next few weeks I did ten minutes, then built up to twelve, and so on. I now practice for twenty to thirty minutes each morning. If you can, it's best to meditate twice a day. Just as we begin each day from a centered place, we wipe away the stress that accumulated throughout the day by practicing again in the late afternoon. Even though I am thoroughly armed with this information, I don't always get a second meditation in. Managing homework, dinner time, and very active sports schedules for my two sons can make afternoons a busy time. I often try to get a few minutes in before they come home from school or get them to meditate with me for a few minutes, but neither are guarantees. For this reason, bringing mindfulness into my entire day is even more important (we'll cover mindfulness in the next chapter).

My meditations begin with sitting in a comfortable position. I believe that comfort is key. There is no rule that you have to sit in a lotus position, or cross-legged at all. Most days I sit in hero pose on two yoga blocks pushed together or on a cushion. You can also sit in a chair with your feet on the floor. If you are short like me, be sure to put a pillow under your feet and bring the floor to you. Another option is to prop yourself up in bed with pillows behind you. I don't recommend laying down because it is much easier to fall asleep, which doesn't count as a meditation; it is considered a nap!

For a long time, I meditated in my closet. I would bring yoga blocks or a zafu cushion in there. Many people like to sit cross-legged on the couch while being supported by the pillows behind them.

It is best to find a position that you can sit in for the duration of your meditation, but if you find yourself really uncomfortable during your practice, feel free to adjust mindfully and then return to your focus. The important takeaway here is that there are no hard and fast rules about how you have to sit to meditate. Try a few ways and stick with what feels right to you.

I always know how long I am going to meditate before I start, and I use a timer that rings with a lovely bell sound. Unless there is some sort of emergency or one of my kids is throwing up, I never stop meditating before the bell rings. And truthfully, that has never happened, thank goodness! I had to train my kids, though. They know that when I am meditating, they are welcome to sit down in my "Zen den" and meditate with me or just enjoy some peace and quiet. Otherwise, they have to wait to talk to me until I am finished. When I started meditating, they would interrupt me to ask questions that could totally wait, but they have gotten used to the routine.

I begin with a body scan to be sure that I am totally relaxed. I start at my head and focus on each body part, all the way down to my toes, as I consciously relax that area of my body.

I then incorporate a bit of mindful breathing, such as counting my breaths, or matching my inhale and exhale. (This will be discussed more in the next section so sit tight.)

Mantra means "an instrument of the mind," and I love incorporating a mantra into my meditation. Just like with mindful breathing, a mantra is used as a focus during your practice. You want to give your mind something to do so that it doesn't go into "story-mode." Examples of story-mode could be your to-do list, your grocery list, plans to redecorate your bedroom, etc. Since we, as humans, are wired to think, we need a focus to be successful in meditation. People are often nervous to try meditation because they think that they have to sit down and magically clear their head of all their thoughts or they aren't meditating successfully. That sounds so *hard* and like a lot of pressure. All you have to do to meditate is to use a focus, and when your mind wanders, come back to it, over and over. There are no goals in meditation, but the purpose is to settle your nervous system and focus on one thing at a time. Concentrating on a mantra makes that easier. It is important to use a mantra that doesn't have much meaning attached to it so that you don't go into story-mode. That is why simple sounds work well, and numbers too.

I always set my timer with an interval at the end, so when the timer goes off I have a few minutes of integration at the end of my practice. This is the part that most people skip, but you want to give your body and mind a chance to integrate all the amazing work you just did. It is wonderful to simply enjoy the stillness and peace for another minute or two, or use this time to set an intention for the rest of the day and say an affirmation or a prayer. If you have ever been to a yoga class, this portion is similar to the last pose of Savasana.

Keep in mind that consistency is key when it comes to meditation. You do not get up from meditation a new person. It is with consistent practice that you begin to see changes happening in your life. In time, you may notice that you are less stressed, sleeping better, are less reactive, and are more productive, just to name a few possible benefits. Others around you may even notice changes before you do. Someone mentioned to me recently that they thought my voice sounded different because I was so much more relaxed.

Five to ten minutes of meditation every day is better than twenty minutes twice a week, but even twenty minutes twice a week is better than nothing. Set yourself up for success by committing to a small amount of time each day that you can build upon. You can compare meditation to taking a shower, brushing your teeth, or cleaning your house. Even if you aren't in the mood, you do it anyway because it is important to have a clean body and a clean home. With meditation, you are clearing stress from your nervous system. It's like dusting from the inside. You don't ever regret taking a shower or brushing your teeth, and you will never regret meditating, either!

If you want to see what meditation feels like, check out my free five-day guided meditation challenge. Every day for five days, I send you a different, eight-minute guided meditation right to your inbox. Visit www.hotmesstomindfulmom.com to register!

In the next chapter, I will cover what you can do if you feel triggered in the moment and you need to reduce stress as quickly as possible.

4

Mindfulness Matters—One Minute Mini-Meditations

"If we are not fully ourselves, truly in the present moment, we miss everything."

—THICH NHAT HANH

My morning meditation practice is an integral part of my routine, but I find that bringing more mindfulness into my entire day takes me to the next level and allows me to fully experience my life as it is happening.

"Mindfulness" is a buzzword today—it's constantly popping up on blogs and magazines, and even being talked about on the news. It means being completely engaged in what you are doing, moment to moment, without judgment.

Whenever I notice that I am distracted, stressed, or bored, I tend to incorporate a mini-meditation, or mindful minute, into my day.

This practice began organically one day when I was sitting at a traffic light. I realized that every time I was stopped at a light—which, living in Houston, is often—I would reach for my phone. I am not sure what important new information I was hoping to learn since it had only been minutes since I last checked it, but I had definitely formed a bad habit.

I also began to notice what other people were doing in their cars at traffic lights, and pretty much everyone I saw was on their phone. I decided to put an end to the madness, if only in my own life.

I started driving with my phone in my purse and using the time spent at lights more mindfully. Instead of scrolling, I began to breathe. I decided to make my breath my new BFF.

Now, each time I stop at a traffic light, I choose a breathing exercise to do. I feel much more relaxed when I arrive places, and it also makes me feel more productive because I am doing something useful with that time.

Some of my favorite mini-meditations include:

Matching my inhale and exhale—As I take a comfortable breath in, expanding my belly 360 degrees as I breathe, as if I'm blowing up a balloon in there. I notice what I count to in my head. It is usually 3, 4, or 5. The different numbers don't matter, you just want the one that feels right to you. I then match my exhale to that number, so if I breathe in to a count of 4, I exhale for a count of 4, and then repeat until the light changes.

Counting my breaths—On the inhale, expanding my belly like I am blowing up a balloon inside of it, I silently count 1, and on the exhale, 2. The next inhale 3, and the next exhale 4, all the way up to 10.

Sweet 16 breathing—Take a deep inhale for a count of 4, hold for a count of 4, exhale for a count of 4, hold for a count of 4. Repeat three times.

Try a one-minute body scan—Notice each body part beginning with your scalp, and consciously relax it as you focus your attention there. In one minute you can focus on your scalp, forehead, cheeks, jaw, tongue, shoulders, chest, stomach, arms, hips, and legs. Focus your attention on each place for about five seconds.

Belly breathing—This is an incredibly simple way to slow down and reset your nervous system. Take a nice long inhale through your nose, almost like you are trying to blow up a balloon that is in your stomach. Hold it for a moment and release slowly through your nose. Repeat five times.

As these mindful minutes began accumulating, I noticed how good they made me feel. I then extended the idea to other areas of my life and began practicing them standing in line at the grocery store, in line at the drive-thru pharmacy, when I felt triggered by my kids, or whenever I felt rushed.

I have coined the phrase "hitting the pause button," because that is exactly what I do. With practice, pausing and breathing have become my new normal when I have extra time, or whenever I feel stressed. It is a much better tactic than flying off the handle and regretting it.

My kids can't help but notice me doing these breathing exercises sometimes. The wonderful result of their perception has been that they now often turn to using their breath as a way to calm down when they are feeling stressed or triggered.

We don't always have extra time in the mornings before school after everyone is dressed, fed, packed up, and teeth are brushed, so I often encourage my kids to do some deep breathing in the car and think of one thing they are grateful for before they hop out in carpool line. I used to get so sad on the days that they would get out of the car in bad moods, or they fought on the way to school, and this makes for a much better routine. I want to send them off to school with smiles, and now I'd say it happens 99 percent of the time.

These mindful minutes bring me back to my calm, peaceful center whenever I need a moment to regroup. One minute of "me" time is often enough to refocus my energy, calm myself when necessary, and help me to feel ready to tackle whatever I am facing with ease and grace.

5

Create a Sacred Space Because You Deserve It!

"Wherever you are—be all there."

—JIM ELLIOTT

Creating a sacred space can be as low-key as choosing your favorite spot on the couch, or as involved as setting up an altar. There are a lot of ways to do it, and all of them are right. Just as there is no wrong way to meditate, there is no wrong place to do it either. Where and when you want to meditate is personal, but it is much more likely that new habits will "stick" if you practice them at a consistent time, in a consistent place.

When I began meditating I would wake up, use the bathroom, and sit right down on the edge of my bathtub. My tub has a step on it and I would put a towel under me and behind me so that I had a cushion for my back and backside. Now that I think about it, I have no idea why I thought that was a good idea! It wasn't that comfortable, and it was a little unusual, but it worked for a while.

A few months later I moved into my closet. It became my quiet little cocoon and I hid in there every morning with the door closed. I began to collect special items on my dresser and before I knew it I had an altar filled with spiritual books, crystals, pictures of loved ones, art from my kids, my vision board, and my worry box (more details on that coming). I transitioned to sitting hero-pose on two yoga blocks pushed together on the floor, and I was cozy and comfortable. That lasted for well over a year.

When I began teaching I turned the front room of my house into my "Zen den" teaching studio. It transformed from a wasted room that nobody used to a sacred space. I found it much easier to decorate a room when your goal is to move furniture out! A fresh coat of creamy paint, adjustable floor cushions, beautiful art, and all my keepsakes and books turned this room into a peaceful and serene haven for my students and myself.

The Zen den is used for my small group classes and private sessions but also daily for my personal meditation practice. I head downstairs between 5:00 and 5:45 a.m. with my two dogs in tow, often lighting a fire in the fireplace on cool mornings, and settling in for my morning spiritual routine.

My routine usually consists of:

- Choosing a crystal to meditate with
- Getting comfortable on my blocks or cushion
- Applying essential oil to my wrists and behind my ears
- Setting my timer and meditating
- Prayer
- Spiritual reading

- Posting an inspirational message on social media
- Writing in my journal

Let me be very clear that none of this is necessary, other than finding a place you are comfortable, setting a timer, and actually meditating. You certainly don't need crystals or oil of any kind. I enjoy creating a routine for myself which encompasses all of these aspects because it makes me feel special. I wake before my household and I like a good forty-five minutes to an hour to start my day. Many people set their alarm fifteen minutes earlier to get a quick meditation in before they start their day. In fact, that is how I encourage my students to start, and that is exactly how I started, with eight minutes a day on the edge of my tub. This routine grew over the course of a few years, and if I am pressed for time, on occasion it can be shortened.

No matter where you meditate or for how long, remember that you are honoring yourself during this time. You are filling up your own cup so that you have more love and joy to share with others that you care about. It is similar to what they say on the airplane before you take off—be sure to put your own oxygen mask on before you help others around you. These five, or ten, or twenty minutes that you spend by yourself each morning do truly fuel you for the rest of the day. When you care for yourself, and begin your day from a calm, centered place, that energy will spread to everyone around you. I love the way that Joseph Campbell puts it: "Your sacred space is where you can find yourself over and over again."

6

Cultivate Gratitude

> *" 'Enough' is a feast."*
> —BUDDHIST PROVERB

Through my work as a meditation and mindfulness teacher, I have found I often end up teaching the very concepts that I need to work on or be reminded of. As I teach them, they solidify even more for me personally. I have found that teaching people to bring more gratitude into their lives always takes them to the next level of their spiritual practice, and is an excellent reminder for me to stay on top of my game as well.

I do feel that the more you practice gratitude, the more the Universe gives you to be grateful for. I began incorporating gratitude into my mindfulness practice after I had been meditating for a while, and I take the time to acknowledge multiple times a day how lucky I am for health, happiness, and the love that surrounds me. I never knew how freeing it would feel to not always be wanting more, because appreciating what I have today makes me feel fulfilled and so very lucky. You

can never be grateful enough. I say "thank you" all day long. Thank you for my beautiful family, for my home, for my dogs, for the education that my children are receiving, for nutritious food, for sunsets, for wonderful friends, for my favorite shows, for inspirational books, for leggings, for my Birkenstocks that I have worn practically every single day for six months, for my runs, for yoga, for a great haircut, for the sound of my boys' giggles, for hugs from my husband who is the greatest person I know on this earth, for my meditations, and for the love I feel for myself. And so much more.

I incorporate gratitude throughout the day, and have several favorite ways to do so.

Thinking of something I am grateful for upon waking is a magnificent way to start the day. Some days it's as simple as being alive, others it may be the sun shining through the window, or my husband snuggled next to me, often with a child between us. Something naturally comes to mind, and I simply say, "thank you, thank you, thank you."

For a long time, I kept a gratitude journal; it's a habit I encourage everyone to incorporate into their routine. My gratitude journal has merged with another journaling technique that I will discuss in another section, but there are amazing journals where you can write one sentence a day. It doesn't have to take a lot of time or feel overwhelming.

If writing isn't your cup of tea, or feels overwhelming, you are creating the same amazing energy in your day when you simply think of something you are grateful for. Don't worry about doing it right or wrong, just do it! Include the big things and the little things. They are all equally as important. Remember, we simply want to be a vibrational match for what we want more of in our life. That can be anything from health to a new lip gloss!

I have an alarm that goes off on my phone every day at 3:00 p.m. to remind me to stop whatever I'm doing, take a deep breath, and spend a minute or two focusing on gratitude.

We practice gratitude as a family as well. We keep a family gratitude journal on our kitchen table, and, at dinner, we go around the table saying something we are grateful for, with one person acting as the scribe.

As I mentioned before, I also encourage my kids to think of something they are grateful for in the morning, often on the way to school. I don't make it a huge deal, it is just part of the everyday routine.

I invite you to start a gratitude practice comprised of whatever feels right to you. Start small with thinking of something you are grateful for in the morning or evening and build from there. Ending my meditations with a moment of gratitude feels really good as well, so try that too!

7

Spiritual Reading—It's Okay to Branch Out from Fiction!

"If you only read the books that everyone else is reading, you can only think what everyone else is thinking."

—HARUKI MURAKAMI

Reading spiritual literature has become a treasured complement to my morning meditation. I feel inspired when I read books such as these that have become favorites on my bookshelves:

- *Holy Shift* by Robert Holden
- *A Year of Miracles and a Return to Love* by Marianne Williamson
- *Miracles Now* and *May Cause Miracles* by Gabby Bernstein
- *A Course in Miracles* from Foundations for Inner Peace
- *How to Practice* by the Dalai Lama
- *An Offering of Leaves* by Ruth Lauer-Manenti

- *The Practice* by Barb Schmidt
- *Soul Centered* by Sarah McLean
- *The Four Agreements* by Don Miguel Ruiz
- *Love Before Fear* by Emily Aube
- *Generation Stressed* by Michele Kambolis
- *Journey to the Heart* by Melody Beattie

I can't wait to add to this list when I get around to reading the stack of books on my bedside table! In addition to those listed, I have read many others for my courses, and even a cursory glance at them on my shelf floods me with gratitude for all I have learned so far on this journey. I feel excited knowing that it is just the beginning; I have so much more knowledge to gain.

Some of these titles are written with the intent that the reader enjoys one or two pages a day, so as not to feel overwhelmed. It is amazing how moved you can feel from just one page of profound writing. This also allows me to easily read one short passage after my morning meditation to seal and close my practice. I don't put pressure on myself to read if I am short on time, but I honestly feel so inspired that I don't want to miss it!

I tend to like reading hard copies or paperbacks of spiritual literature because I can underline and turn down pages. The only problem is that the books are a mess to lend out!

It can also be fun to bond with friends and loved ones over a beautiful book. Consider starting a book club, or even having a reading partner that you can discuss a book or passage with. It is always so interesting to get someone else's take on a book. This is a great way to stay in touch with someone that you care about that you don't get to see much, because this can be done on the phone or via Skype over a mug of your favorite hot tea.

8

Never Stop Learning

"If it's both terrifying and amazing then you should definitely pursue it."
—ERADA

I was definitely in a new-mom fog for a few years (or eight). I lived in my own bubble of meals, diapers, preschool, milestones, *Bob Books*, and Little League. I literally had no idea what was going on in the world around me. My husband was in charge of telling me if anything major happened in the world, such as a war breaking out. I have never really been much of a TV person so the news was never on, and I was too busy reading *Mouse Makes Words* to get involved with the paper, even online. It was such an egotistical way to live—if it didn't concern my immediate existence I just didn't have time for it. Not to mention it was embarrassing to be in public and have a current event brought up and have no clue what anyone was talking about. I started asking my husband for briefings on current events in the car on the way to parties so that I didn't appear as clueless as I was.

It takes a tremendous amount of physical and emotional energy to stay at home with your kids. I wouldn't trade it for anything, but I worked *hard* for those eight years solely in my home. It was also an insular existence, and I only really came into contact with my family and other moms doing the same things that I was.

When I began my teaching certification program my world expanded. Parts of my brain came out of hibernation and I loved learning again. I felt challenged in a different way and I appreciated how this new knowledge was adding to my own meditation practice. Everyone I met in my program was incredibly unique and opened my eyes to new ideas. I felt invigorated and more passionate in all areas of my life.

Through my studies, I not only learned about the collective consciousness, how everything in the Universe is connected, but truly began to feel its existence. Our energy affects the people and the world around us. This also made me want to learn more about what was going on beyond my zip code.

I began to stay abreast of current events. Not that I would go head to head in a debate about anything, but I was at least familiar and had a bit to add to a conversation here and there. I am truly grateful for my daily email subscription to the *Skimm*. It is kind of funny that I first learned about it from reading *US Weekly*, (my Friday brain candy), but it has been a game-changer for me. Every morning I get an email about domestic and international current events, and everything is explained for news newbies like myself. It is awesome!

The stack of books next to my bed is so high it teeters. I have always been an avid fiction reader, but the topics I enjoy now range from meditation to self-help to Kundalini yoga. I simply can't get enough. I am not just an active participant in conversations now, but

I lead many of them. I could talk about meditation and spirituality all day long. My style is pretty down to earth, and my goal is to make everyone I talk to feel comfortable discussing these topics.

If you had asked me six years ago whether I would ever meditate, let alone teach and inspire others to meditate, I would have looked at you like you had two heads. It wasn't even on my radar yet, so who's to say what else is coming my way. I am so much more open-minded and curious now. Once I started learning again, it just made me want more.

Is there something you have thought about studying but you never did because of time constraints? Is it hard to admit you are interested in a topic that is different than what your contemporaries are into? Don't let that stop you. Go for it!

I am now learning about crystal healing, Ayurveda, and essential oils, which sound kind of "out there" to many people, but I couldn't care less. It is my time and energy. I encourage everyone to find one topic to learn about, and it doesn't have to be academic. Studying and practicing in any fashion keeps us connected to the world around us and broadens our horizons. Maybe it is food, health, or fashion that interests you. Maybe child development, psychology, or graphic design. The sky is the limit.

What have you always wanted to learn about? We are so lucky to live in a day and age where knowledge is at our fingertips, so go for it, even if it is simply reading an article or blog post in your minute or two of downtime a day.

9

Cut Yourself Some Slack

"Do not tolerate disrespect—even from yourself."
—UNKNOWN

I was talking to a high school friend on the phone recently and I had a bonding moment with her that honestly took me by surprise. I truly adore this woman. She is one of those fun-loving, tell-it-like-it-is people who are amazing to be around, and if we lived in the same city I know we would be connected at the hip. The conversation started out rather superficially but quickly turned into a deeper one than either of us expected.

We were actually comparing boob jobs. Years ago I would have told you that having cosmetic surgery as a mom was selfish. What if something unthinkable happened on the table? I often said that it would never be worth it, but that was before I wanted elective surgery and I changed my tune.

For months, every time I looked in the mirror I pictured what I would look like with perfect boobs like the ones I had before my

pregnancies. I became obsessed with the mental image. I began to look at other women who had even obvious breast implants with jealousy, and I envisioned how I would look with tight, perky breasts once more. I tortured myself like this until I decided that life was just too short not to have breast augmentation surgery. I had to accept the fact that I really wanted to do it, and love myself enough to honor this desire. I simply didn't judge myself for it.

My surgery and recovery were uneventful, and I felt immense gratitude for that. For a few weeks I looked like a porn star due to the swelling, but when it finally went down I looked exactly how I'd hoped. Not too big, not too small, and nothing that anyone would notice unless they knew to look.

My friend commented on the crazy fact that people can change their bodies so drastically in a matter of hours. It was so easy. One day we had deflated boobs, and the next day we didn't. And with that, I burst into tears.

I had been feeling nostalgic at the time for my boys' younger years. I found myself standing in front of their baby pictures in our hallway for long periods, simply staring at their adorable baby and toddler faces. I truly do love every stage of childhood, and I wouldn't trade the conversations we have now even for a toothless grin, but occasionally I just want to go back for a moment. I want to kiss their damp baby curls when I pick them up from their crib after a nap. I want to push a stroller and coo at them, because now they run so fast I can hardly keep up.

As my tears fell, words came out of my mouth that I had never expressed. I honestly didn't even know they existed in my heart, and I was just as surprised to hear them as my friend was. "I want to do it again. I want to do it again as me NOW. I am so much better now. I want to do it without drama. I know what I am doing and I like myself so much more now."

Our conversation ended, but my words haunted me for days.

I truly feel like I woke up around thirty-six years of age. My spiritual journey began when I realized that growth was possible for me. I didn't need to emulate anyone else, in fact quite the opposite. I needed to find out who I really was. It was time to come into my own. I didn't even feel like I knew myself. I presented a secure front, or at least tried to, but underneath that façade, I was an insecure mess.

I fluctuated between being pissed at myself for wasting so much time and energy on the wrong things, like mom drama and who was carrying which designer handbag, and working to forgive myself. Eventually, I had to give myself a stern talking-to in order to quiet my ego.

I said it over and over until I believed it. "Cut yourself some slack. You are doing the best you can, and you always have. Even the silly things you have done and said were done with good intentions at the time. You didn't set out to screw up! Everyone makes mistakes, and those are the experiences that help us to learn, grow, and become better people."

Instead of begrudging the painful and embarrassing experiences, I began to reframe them and feel grateful because they did help me grow. If I hadn't learned from them, I may still be trying to one-up other moms with my kids' test scores and how many goals they scored on the soccer field.

The time that it took to navigate and overcome my emotional pain certainly highlights the contrast between making physical changes and emotional ones. With a good dose of anesthesia, two bags of silicone, and a few stitches, your physical body is changed for good. If only it were that easy to grow emotionally and mentally.

Our internal landscape cannot change as quickly as the external one. Even though I love the way my body looks since I had my

surgery, it is nothing compared to the changes I've made in my psyche. I am much more beautiful on the inside. I feel deeper, have more compassion, more gratitude, and more faith. I can honestly say that I am pretty great. Not perfect by any means, but who is?

The biggest test of my newfound self-acceptance comes when I mess up in front of other people. Because I am a spiritual teacher, many people think that I never yell or think a bad thought. I am still human, and even if I try to keep my cool most of the time, there are occasions that I don't and it sucks when I have an audience.

I remember the day that I raised my voice at one of my kids just as they were going into a tutoring session. My son was being disrespectful and it triggered me. Instead of pausing and taking a deep breath, I promptly reprimanded him. The tutor was in the other room and she definitely heard. I immediately felt bad and apologized to my son and squeezed him to death in a bear hug. It's funny, the less you yell at your kids, the worse it feels when it happens. I usually practice what I teach, like taking deep breaths and responding instead of reacting, but once in a blue moon I just react in a way that makes me feel terrible. After I apologized to Adam, I then began to panic that I looked like a total fraud in front of his tutor. My ego completely took over and went crazy. Here I am, teaching others how not to do exactly what I just did! She had mentioned wanting to come to me to learn to meditate and I went into a downward spiral of doubt that she would never want to know. And then I had to STOP. THE. MADNESS.

The mistakes that I beat myself up over will not be my last. I will put my foot in my mouth dozens more times: I will forget to invite someone to a birthday party, I will yell at my kids again, and I will disappoint my loved ones and myself. The difference will be my attitude. I will be sorry, and I may even have regrets, but I will cut myself some slack. Instead of seeing stupidity I will recognize growth. I will learn, internalize, and soar. I will model for my kids that we all make mistakes. I will assure them that these mistakes do not define us; what we learn from them does.

10

Have a Running Buddy

"Friendship is not a big thing . . . it's a million little things."
—UNKNOWN

I am pretty obsessed with my husband. I call him my gift from the Universe. Mark is the most supportive, understanding, and encouraging person I know. He is an amazing father, a hard worker, and the life of the party. Saying Mark is outgoing is an understatement. He can make friends with anyone, anywhere. He is caring and performs random acts of kindness all the time. I have learned more about being a good person from him than anyone else in my life. I knew Mark was meant for me on our third date—I had never dated anyone where I felt truly accepted for just being me. I had dated guys where I said what I thought they wanted to hear, and I vowed never to do that again. Mark is truly my partner in every sense of the word—but he is not my running buddy. I don't hide anything from Mark, and I can truly talk to him about anything under the sun, but occasionally you just need a girlfriend.

Mark and I share many of the same interests, such as our kids and dogs (obviously), and enjoy doing things together like going to the movies, taking walks, and talking about everything under the sun over a glass of wine for him, and a seltzer for me. We support each other's work and encourage constant growth in our lives. I am incredibly proud of the business that Mark has built over the past twenty years, and he is equally as proud of the business that I am growing. He sees how fulfilling it is, and celebrates the transformation he sees in me. Mark is open-minded to a certain extent. He is all for me bringing spirituality into my life, but he isn't really interested in bringing it into his own. The reason this works is because I have never pressured Mark for a second to do something just because I do it.

I knew Mark really didn't want to meditate when he turned down offers infused with some pretty hefty incentives. When I first launched my business I was desperate to practice leading a few guided meditations before I taught actual students. It would have been so easy to practice on Mark after the kids went to bed. I put forth an irresistible offer, or so I thought—for every guided meditation that Mark allowed me to lead him through, I would give him a sexual favor after we were done. Who would say no? Relax for a few minutes, and then *really* relax. Well, he never took me up on the offer, which made it crystal clear that he really didn't want to meditate. I have never asked him again. I figure when he's ready, he will let me know.

Many people say that it is good for couples to share the same hobbies so they spend more time together. That may work for some people, but honestly, in my marriage, I have found the opposite to be true. Mark loves playing cards and golf. Given a hall pass, I want to go for a run or take a yoga class. We both feel that we benefit as

a couple and a family when we have time away from it all and feel rejuvenated when we come back home. People often ask me if I mind that Mark is out one or two nights a week playing cards. They say they would never let their husbands do that. How a marriage works is very personal. I never mind Mark taking a night or two away during the week because every minute that he is home, he is 100 percent on. The kids wait by the door with baseball gloves or a football in hand when the garage door opens, and Mark usually doesn't make it in the door unless he has a catch outside first. He is bike riding on the weekends, coaching their teams, and usually winning our board game marathons. And honestly, having a night or two to myself after the kids go to bed to catch up on work, write, or to get in bed and read quietly is nice. The time Mark and I spend apart only tends to make us enjoy the time we have together more. For us, it works, and there is no guilt. It gets harder and harder to leave during the week, as homework and sports schedules ramp up, but if I want to have dinner with a friend it works both ways. I don't feel bad about taking a night out every once in a while.

Connecting with like-minded individuals who share the same interests is important. I have different "running buddies" for different areas of my life. Sharing experiences makes them more fun and meaningful.

I have a few friends that are my actual running buddies. I love running with them because it turns exercise into social time as well. It's not always easy to squeeze in time with friends, but exercising with them is like getting a two-for-one. It is amazing how much personal stuff can come up when you run with someone often. We have a saying: "What is said on a run, stays on the run."

I also have my spiritual running buddies. These are the friends with whom I talk meditation and mindfulness. We share stories about our transformations and "aha!" moments. I have met many of these wonderful people through my classes, and we support and encourage each other as we take our gifts out into the world. We swap business ideas, give honest feedback, and laugh a lot. They are spread all over the country, and I feel blessed that I have met these amazing people.

My life would not be the same without my two besties who get me through each day. We commiserate about all the mommy things and girlie things, and are there for each other through thick and thin. I met both of these women way back when. Jamie I met at college freshman orientation, and Misha as soon as I graduated. They have seen me go through every stage of my adult life, and they still love me—that says a lot! Our friendships have survived moves across the country and the world, and frankly, nothing could break us up. I trust these ladies with my life.

Where would I be without my actual sisters, Amy, Susan, and Stephanie? My two older sisters and my identical twin lived through the same mess of a childhood, and somehow we all turned out to be upstanding members of our community, with successful careers and loving families. It is somewhat of a miracle! There are no secrets among us, only unconditional love.

All of these people fill different roles in my life. I treasure and value each and every one of them. Even though I adore spending time alone, I am not a loner. These relationships fuel me. My only hope is that I do just as good a job offering love and support to them as these people do for me.

We all need a safe person to vent to once in a while to unload our worries and sadness. Nobody is happy all the time. I tried to be, and I just ended up ignoring everything until the stress built up in my body to the point of combustion. We have got to let it out, but choosing the right time and place to do so is critical. We don't need to announce our deepest, darkest secrets to twenty colleagues over drinks after work, or spill our guts to random moms at a school event. Instead, we need to find a few trusted confidantes who will be there for us with wise words and warm hugs.

Running buddies can be like-minded souls that you have common interests with, or simply amazing people that make you feel safe and cared for. No matter what, be sure you have one or two people in your life whom you can trust completely and that the relationship is mutual. There should never be one person doing all the unloading, all the time. Taking turns is part of the fun!

11

Honor Yourself

"You are braver than you believe, stronger than you seem,
smarter than you think, and loved more than you know."

—A.A. MILNE

I lived for years saying "yes" to everything because I never wanted to disappoint anyone, but the more mindful I became, the more self-aware I became as well. I began to notice that I actually had opinions and feelings, and I didn't have to be self-conscious or insecure when it came to sharing them.

My teacher and mentor, Sarah McLean, talks about understanding your "yums" and your "yucks." There is no need for me to find my own words that mean the same thing—hers are just perfect.

When you begin to pay attention to your body you will notice that it sends you signals you can use to assist in making nourishing decisions for yourself, like saying no to something that is going to send you over the edge. Our minds often get confused, but our bodies never do. When something is a "heck yeah" or a no-brainer, our body may send us signals, like feelings of joy, excited butterflies, a smile, or the feeling when you want to pump your fist in the air and scream, "YES!"

But when something is a "please God, help me get out of this," or an "I think I just came down with the flu," then your body may send you a signal, like sweaty palms, shortness of breath, sweating, stomach cramps, anxiety, and stress.

These signals are your own personal SOS code. You get one of these and you let your body guide you to safety.

I tell my students to say "yes" when you really mean it, and learn how to say "no" nicely when you don't. It can feel hard at first, but trust me, it gets easier. We only have a limited amount of free time in our lives, and we have to use it for things that are truly calling to us, and are a "heck yeah." I have found that the build-up in our minds prior to saying no is worse than actually saying it. I learned this lesson when it came to finding a place to volunteer in the community.

It took me forever to find the right place to volunteer. Serving the community is important to me, but for a while, I just couldn't find the right fit. I began volunteering at my children's school, which seemed like an obvious place to start. I realized that I loved doing activities where I had contact with my kids during the day, like serving lunch or reading in their classrooms, but I didn't enjoy being in the PTO. I am really grateful that there are people that do because they keep the school going, but I am just not one of them. Planning fundraisers and events at school didn't fulfill me at all, so I served lunch, but I started saying "no" to everything else.

I then tried volunteering at Texas Children's Hospital in Houston, which is world-renowned, and we are fortunate to have it in our backyard should we ever need it. It has an incredible volunteer network, so I had high hopes for the placement. I love kids, and they do oodles of good there, so it seemed like a perfect fit. But it wasn't. Many people love volunteering there, but I always felt like I was in no-man's land, and I left feeling depleted and bored. The short spurts that I spent with kids were wonderful but there was way too much downtime for me, and I soon realized that it wasn't a match. Instead of feeling like a failure, I became more determined to find the right place, and I finally did.

Dress for Success became volunteer heaven for me. In case you aren't familiar with the organization, Dress for Success is a "global not-for-profit organization that promotes the economic independence of disadvantaged women by providing professional attire, a network of support, and the career development tools to help women thrive in work and in life." I volunteered four hours a month as a personal shopper. Working with two women per shift, I helped them find the perfect interview suit, a blouse, purse, shoes, and scarf. Even more importantly than how they look when they leave is how they felt—like they could tackle the world. Nothing beats seeing the way the women smile when they look in the mirror and feel transformed. I was filled with love for these beautiful souls and this amazing organization every single time I went. I also loved the feeling of camaraderie among the volunteers and the warm staff.

I knew it was the right place for me because I got a "yum" every other Monday morning when I get dressed, and that is saying a lot because I had to shed my usual uniform of leggings and a sweatshirt for business attire. I was not thinking about my to-do list, or what else I could be doing while I was there. Instead, I was excited to be a small part of someone turning her life around.

My newest volunteer endeavor is training my tiny and adorable nine-pound Shih Tzu, Lacy, to be a therapy dog. We are working hard to pass the test because spending more time with her, and allowing her to brighten even more lives outside of our home, feels like a perfect fit for the next stage of my volunteer life.

I have also learned to nourish myself socially. I have become a tad choosier about what I am leaving my kids and husband for. There were many times in the past that I went out multiple nights a week because I didn't want to be left out of a plan. I hated the idea of people having fun without me (I had a total case of FOMO), which goes to show just how insecure I was. But many of those times I sat at the table wishing that I was home tucking my kids into bed. I love Moms' Night Out as much as the next mom in the carpool line, but I just don't need as many as I used to. I have become a bit of a homebody, and I realize that the days of my kids wanting me to snuggle with them in bed each night are numbered. Eventually, they won't want me to, so I want to soak up every Eskimo kiss and back tickle that I can. Unless my body gives me a "hell yes" when I get that email or text to go out, I pass until next time.

Begin to pay attention to your "yums and yucks," and honor yourself by saying "yes" only when you mean it!

12

Spend Time in Nature

"Some old fashioned things like fresh air and sunshine are hard to beat."
—LAURA INGALLS WILDER

I moved to Houston in August of 1998, right after I graduated from George Washington University and backpacked through Europe on $20 a day—no joke. That included hotel, food, and activities. If we had a private bathroom in our hotel room we were living large, and I literally survived in Greece on salad and falafel from a stand for two weeks straight. But it was amazing in every way, and made me appreciate my 35th birthday trip to Europe with my husband even more. Nothing beat being in Italy and being able to order whatever I wanted for dinner. Pizza and pasta? Yes, please!

I remember walking from the parking lot to my first job at Enron in downtown Houston with sweat literally dripping from every square inch of my body. I vividly remember wearing a dorky purple sweater set, wide-legged black pants, and scuffed black flats my first

day and saying to myself, "It will never be worse than this. This is as bad as it will ever be."

Fortunately, it did cool off around Thanksgiving. I truly appreciated the "winter" months of December and January and spent every moment outside that I could, most likely rollerblading at the time. Remember rollerblades? I was terrible!

As much I would love to be walking on a beach in California, or hiking the red rocks of Sedona every day, it is just not happening. I have learned to appreciate what I can get and to be mindful whenever I am outside.

I now leave my phone on the counter when I take my dogs for a walk, and I have swapped scrolling Facebook for looking at the shapes in the clouds. I notice the way the breeze feels on my skin, smell the freshly cut grass, and stop to admire beautiful flowers.

It is important for me to get outside every day, even if it is just for a quick walk around the block or to sip tea on my back porch. On nice days I may write outside, and reading in my backyard is on the top of my list if I ever have free time on a sunny day.

Whenever I am in need of inspiration, in terms of work or personal situations, somehow spending a few minutes outside seems to broaden my perspective and give me a fresh spin on things. If I ever feel stuck, the first thing I do is head outdoors.

I encourage you to find some way to be outside each day, even for a few short minutes. Walk the kids to school, drink your coffee outside on your back step or by an open window, eat a meal outside on nice days, or even stand outside while you are on the phone.

I have also started planning walking dates with friends. Instead of spending more time at Starbucks, we meet for a walk. We get time to catch up and be in nature, with no calories!

13

Get Grounded

"We can't direct the wind, but we can adjust the sails."
—THOMAS MONSON

We all have days where we feel a bit out of control. No matter how much we meditate and how mindful we are, they still come, just hopefully not as often. Our kids, spouses, partners, and other loved ones also have harder days occasionally, and it is easy to feed off this energy.

I have found that with the right tools it is easier to get out of a funk and get grounded when I need to. The following techniques work for me, and may be a good starting point for you, or perhaps a springboard for you to come up with some of your own ways to reclaim your positive energy when life feels overwhelming.

Water—Water is very grounding, so hop in a nice warm bath with Epsom salts or drink some hot tea.

Exercise—There is something about going on a run that lifts my spirits no matter what is going on. Yoga is also amazing for me, but

it is getting the body—and any negative energy—moving that does the trick. Walk, bike, hike, dance . . . just get moving.

Spending time with my pets—Sometimes I would give anything for my pets to be able to talk, and then there are times when I am so glad they can't! Laying on the floor and connecting with my dogs is extremely calming for me. If you don't have a pet, ask a neighbor if you can borrow theirs for a few minutes. I am sure they would love the extra attention. Some shelters will even allow you to borrow dogs for a few hours to take on hikes or walks.

Journaling—It is amazing how ideas and feelings flow when you allow yourself to focus on them. Let it all out with your pen.

Prayer—Sometimes I simply ask the Universe for guidance and to help me see a situation in a new way. Don't be afraid to ask for help.

Extra meditations—My morning meditation keeps me on a pretty even keel, but sometimes I need a little booster during the day. Even three minutes can do the trick.

Reiki—I am Reiki 2 certified, which means I can practice on myself and others. This type of energy work can help tremendously. Ask around—a friend may be certified and willing to work on you for extra practice.

Time in nature—A walk around the block or sitting in the sun in my backyard can be incredibly restorative. A minute or two is all it takes.

Grounding crystals—I am very sensitive to crystal energy and I often work with smoky quartz or black tourmaline for grounding. Give them a try! Their natural beauty is often enough to lift my spirits.

Exhaling—When we exhale we can let out all the stress we feel. We then have the opportunity to decide what we are bringing in on the next inhale. Will it be the same stress and anxiety, or will it be calm and peace? The choice is yours.

Reading—I love getting lost in a good book. It is a great way to take a break from whatever is going on. After a chapter or two, I am usually ready to dive back into my day.

Singing at the top of my lungs—I have a horrible voice, but I love to sing. When I am alone in my car I will belt out tunes like "Blank Space" by Taylor Swift, "Super Bass" by Nicki Minaj, or even old-school "Leather and Lace" by Stevie Nicks. If anyone heard me I would be mortified!

Cooking—If I haven't been taking care of myself and eating nutritious food, it shows in my energy levels. When I feel rundown or like I haven't been prioritizing my health as much, I will spend a few hours in the kitchen preparing food for the next few days that I can grab and feel good about eating.

Connecting—There are weeks that my husband and I are like two ships passing in the night because we are often in two different directions in the afternoon and evening with our kids, shuttling them to and from their activities. After a long day, we often fall into bed with a quick hug and kiss and without a real conversation. If this happens a few too many times it makes me feel needy, and I know that it is time to connect in an authentic way (like having sex and a great conversation afterward).

Girl time—I have been working very hard to build my business over the past few years. I went from being a stay-at-home mom to

a working mom, and my social time has been cut drastically. I love what I do, and wouldn't change it for the world, but I need to be sure I don't lose all my social connections. It can feel difficult to maintain balance in this area, so at times I must prioritize my friendships. I'll squeeze in a coffee date or a walk, even if it means staying up late after the kids go to bed once in a while to catch up on a bit of work.

Sleep—This is a BIG one. The amount of sleep that a person runs on varies from individual to individual. Some people require nine to ten hours, while others feel that they function well on five to six. I would say that seven hours is my magic number. If I go a night or two getting more like six, I can definitely feel it the next day.

It is important to understand what makes you feel stronger and more grounded when you feel yourself on the brink of exhaustion, dealing with negative energy, or your energy is low. Try to have some items on hand (Epsom salts, a journal, a good book, etc.) if you know they are your go-to solution.

14

Mindful Eating

"When walking, walk. When eating, eat."
—ZEN PROVERB

One of the hardest areas of my life to incorporate mindfulness has been the way I eat. I have been a fast eater my entire life, but having babies took it to a whole new level. I learned how to hold a baby, balance the bottle, and somehow eat at the same time. For years, I had more meals at my kitchen counter than my table, and always standing up. The typical "kid food" I was serving to my boys wasn't that tempting. I inhaled my food so quickly that I wasn't ever sure how much I ate, or if I even enjoyed it.

I will never forget the night that my husband and I first went out to dinner without our kids, who were very young at the time. Even though we were alone, the habit of rushing through our meals was so ingrained in us that we did it anyway. We ate in about three minutes, and, all of a sudden, I looked up from my plate to see the couple at the table next to us was staring at us with their mouths hanging open. We must have looked like total pigs inhaling like that!

As the kids got older, meals became much more relaxing, but old habits die hard, and I hadn't made much progress in slowing down when I ate. It became clear that better habits were not going to magically take hold in my life, so I had to put some effort into becoming more mindful of how I eat. It has taken a few months, but I have definitely observed progress.

The first thing I incorporated into my routine was doing a quick body scan before eating. I close my eyes, take a deep breath, and notice if I am holding any tension in my body before a meal. Self-awareness can bring on some unusual revelations, and I realized that I always had an anxious feeling before I took my first bite of food. I honestly don't know if it had to do with the choices I was making, or if I felt pressed for time, but it didn't seem like a good thing. By taking a mindful moment to breathe and calm my body down, I began eating with a sense of peace and calm.

I didn't grow up saying Grace, but it is a lovely tradition. Our food doesn't simply appear on the table. Nature is responsible for a large part, and there are many people who help bring nutritious food to us. Everyone from the farmers to the truck drivers, to the people at the grocery store and whoever prepared the meal have all done something to make it possible for us to eat. It feels good to take a moment to express gratitude for all these moving parts coming together and making it seem effortless for us to have a meal. After my body scan, I quickly acknowledge Mother Nature and everyone else who made this possible. I then take it a step further and bless the actual food. I heard one of my mentors, Gabby Bernstein, say she does this, and I adopted it. I simply say, "I love my food, and my food loves me." I do this in the hopes that if I send love to my food it will do its best to nourish me and keep me healthy. I like to play it safe!

My kids think this routine is weird. They always ask me what I am doing, no matter how many times they watch me. I simply tell them that I am "calming myself before I eat, and being grateful for my food." I would like to start having them participate in at least the gratitude portion. I want to encourage them to spend more time appreciating where their food comes from, and understanding that it doesn't magically appear. It takes money, time, hard work, and nature to make it all possible. I guess I know what we're working on next.

15

Don't Forget to Play

When my kids were little I used to spend hours playing on the floor with them. That was basically our whole agenda some days—tummy time, reading books, and walks. Then, slowly, life started getting more complicated. They had playdates and activities, lunches and snacks that needed to be packed for school, homework came into play, and sports took over our lives. Somehow the playtime began to disappear. I started working part-time and often felt like I was running on a hamster wheel. There were days I was just trying to make it through to get dinner on the table before I collapsed into bed exhausted. Those were the days that I lost the joy.

I didn't even know there was another way until I was on the other side of the chaos. I didn't want to feel like I was in the trenches of motherhood; I wanted to actually enjoy my day-to-day life.

I realized that I could continue to be neurotic about my house being neat every minute of the day, which meant that I never sat down because I was constantly cleaning and organizing, or I could ease up on the house and savor special moments with my family, creating memories and appreciating each other's company.

It all started one day when I caught myself being anal. My son asked me to play a game with him and I started to say I would come-over as soon as I finished folding the laundry. I stopped and checked in with myself. What was I doing? My son actually wanted to play with me. Did it really matter if the laundry wasn't folded for another thirty minutes? Of course not! So, for the first time, I walked away from a household task in order to play. You know what? The world did not fall apart, and neither did my house.

After sitting on the floor that first time to play backgammon and chat with my son about our day, it got easier to find balance. I prioritized playtime again. It may not be for hours, but I try to find ten to fifteen minutes every day to do something that is purely fun with the kids. It may be a quick game of gin, hangman at the kitchen counter, or a short basketball game outside.

These days, not having quality time to enjoy my kids bothers me more than the pile of laundry.

16

Get Your Groove On

"My taste in music ranges from 'you need to listen to this' to 'I know, please don't judge me.'"

—*A SOUTHERN FAIRYTALE* **BLOG**

Some days I am in the mood for sweatpants and UGGs, and others ankle-length jeans and ballet flats. It's nice to have options, and I'm glad that my closet represents lots of shopping mood swings. Music is like that for me as well. Some days I need Top 40, others "hippy dippy" meditation music, and just like a good TBT on Facebook, sometimes I want 10,000 Maniacs and Sting, just like in my college days.

Fortunately, my iTunes account has just as much commitment-phobia as my closet. Even though I am not the biggest music buff out there (like my best friend from high school, who owned every album the day it came out and instantly knew the words to every song—I still can't figure out how she did that), I appreciate how it can relax me when I need it to, or pump me up when I need a boost.

I have music I like to cook to, run to, drive to, work to, and chant. The best is when I can find a song that my whole family likes and we have impromptu dance parties. Usually, it's the new Top 40 song that is being blasted in my bathroom during my kids' shower time at night. They have gone to bed late some nights because we just keep dancing. Those are the times when I had to send parental judgment out the door and just have fun.

My kids LOVE to play DJ. My older son hijacks my phone and picks songs in the car. This is the best mood booster I have found. Any day that he wakes up on the wrong side of the bed and is a little moody in the morning, I tell him to pick a song to listen to on the way to school, and he perks right up. Next thing you know we are all singing along, and even though they would never admit it, my boys know the words to lots of my meditation music chants and they totally sing them without even meaning to. I love it!

Sing-offs are another great activity when we arrive somewhere early. Seatbelts are clicked off in the parking lot (usually before baseball), one kid picks a song, and we all belt it out at the top of our lungs and dance in our seats. I am not sure who has more fun, me or the kids.

Take one night after the kids go to sleep and play around with a few playlists. Create one for workouts, one for quiet time, one for driving, one as a good mood booster, and one for cooking. There are days that the thought of making dinner has me gagging, so the music really helps!

17

Respect a Schedule

"A good laugh and a long sleep are the two best cures for anything."
—IRISH PROVERB

I remember the days when my kids were babies and toddlers and we adhered to a 7:00 p.m. bedtime for them. I started dinner around 5:00 in the evening and bath time shortly after because it was a great activity to fill some time. A few snuggles and stories later that sound machine went on, ocean waves lulled the boys to sleep, and it was finally time to relax. My husband and I had a few hours to spend either together or apart binge watching TV or reading. I am trying to remember if I actually appreciated those downtime-filled evenings enough as they were happening. Probably not.

These days, I'd like to say the boys go to bed at 9:00, but most nights it's closer to 9:30 or even 9:45 by the time they are settled and ready for the final round of hugs. By then I am exhausted! Even though they are at school all day, I always run out of time and seem to have a list of things I am supposed to do after they go to bed—

write a newsletter or blog post, finish editing a chapter, confirming appointments with clients, not to mention catching up with a friend, reading for fun, watching a show, or maybe talking to my husband. There is absolutely no way that I can do all of that and adhere to the 10:30 bedtime I like to keep. I have to make choices and prioritize.

Some nights, if a new episode of a favorite show is on demand, it takes priority over everything else. I have very few shows I care about watching, but nothing can keep me from the ones I like. Other nights I really feel like I need to get some work done, but I have to be realistic about what I can do in about forty-five minutes so I still have a bit of time to wind down before bed.

I should be clear that this is the goal. If I am really on a roll accomplishing a task I may stay up a bit later, but I always pay the price the next day. It just isn't good for me to skimp on sleep, so I do my best to honor my bedtime.

I am very much a morning person. I can hop out of bed for a meditation or workout easily if I have gotten a decent night's sleep, hence the (mostly) strict bedtime. I really need that time in the morning before the rest of my household gets up, so if I sleep in I pay the price in other ways. I hate that rushed feeling in the morning, and I avoid it at all costs.

I am also trying to adhere to more of a schedule when it comes to social media. I adore social media. I find incredible inspiration online and truly enjoy connecting with other like-minded souls on various sites. I find it relaxing and fun, but if I am not careful it can be a huge time suck in my life.

My goal is to be off completely by 9:00 each night, and not to log on in the morning until after I have meditated and done a little spiritual reading. I find that I am much less distracted in my meditations when I do not look at emails and social media beforehand. I am

also attempting to stay on social media twice a day for a maximum of fifteen minutes at a time instead of letting thirty minutes or an hour pass without even realizing where the time went.

In regards to my schedule and my life, some days are better than others. I do my best, but life happens. Flexibility is as much of a gift as a perfectly scheduled day.

18

Bite-Sized Journaling

"We do not learn from experience . . . we learn from reflecting on experience."
—JOHN DEWEY

When I hear the word "journal" I immediately imagine trips to Papyrus to pick out beautifully crafted books filled with raw-edged paper and single-spaced lines. Then I envision stolen moments curled up on the couch with a soft blanket, hot tea, and a gel roller pen. As lovely as that picture is in my imagination, the reality feels different for me. The blank pages used to freak me out because I panicked that I wouldn't have enough to say to fill them. Now, I am so used to typing on a keyboard that my hand cramps when I write a lot, which can be a total deal-breaker when journaling. Talk about a buzzkill.

Journaling is the one part of my spiritual practice that took forever to feel good to me. I liked the idea of it, but I ended up feeling inadequate. I am certain there is a reason for this if a therapist analyzed the situation, but I am okay admitting that I just wasn't the

journaling type for a long time. I have a lot to say to the Universe, but I felt most comfortable doing it in prayer or by writing a short note in my Worry Box.

My Worry Box sits on a shelf in my Zen den (aka my teaching studio). It's the place that I put notes to the Universe when I am seeking guidance on an issue or manifesting a desired outcome from a situation. I enjoy this practice, and since I believe the Universe has my back, all I have to do is ask for help and it will come in one form or another. I am sometimes specific and sometimes general, but I am always open to being shown a completely different solution than I thought would come. It usually takes a few days, but a resolution of some kind seems to reveal itself when I am open to noticing the signs given to me. Answers often come in the form of a deep inner-knowing that I didn't have before. I am suddenly so sure of what I need to do or say.

On one of my many searches on Amazon (Prime is the best thing that ever happened to me) I came across a slew of journals called 5 Minute Journals, and I was intrigued. I was game because it seemed that here was absolutely no way I could fail—and I really did want to give journaling a try in some way.

I ordered the one with the cover I liked the best (a taupe linen to match my bathroom), and decided that even a few lines a day was better than nothing—at least this way I didn't have to feel self-inflicted pressure about journaling anymore. I will give anything a shot at least once.

It turns out that the tiny bit of journaling I did each day became a treasured part of my routine, and I now encourage all my students to incorporate it into their days as well. It offers the perfect amount of mindfulness in the morning and evening without feeling like you added a big task to your day.

I keep my journal next to my toothbrush on my bathroom counter. I always brush my teeth first thing in the morning, and the last thing at night, so the timing coincides perfectly.

In the morning, the journal prompts me to write three things I am grateful for. This is wonderful, but I changed how I do it slightly. I choose one thing I am grateful for each day and write three sentences about it. Doing so allows me to delve a bit deeper into my feelings, and I like that. Next, I write three things I hope happen that day, and lastly, an affirmation for the day.

In the evening I am prompted to write three amazing things that did happen that day and one thing that I could have done better. I use this time to reflect upon my day and think about what I experienced, and the lessons I learned. What can I improve upon, and what can I celebrate?

I spend approximately two minutes, tops, in the morning and evening. It is just enough to make me think, hope, and reflect. If you were contemplating starting a journaling practice but it felt like too much of a commitment, this is the perfect way to take baby steps and try it out.

19

Just Say "No" to Drama

"Do not let the behavior of others destroy your inner peace."
—DALAI LAMA

I was talking to a friend during an early morning workout about the drama that some people stir up, and she said something that made me incredibly jealous. She said that it was an innate quality in her family to stay away from drama. She was always taught by her parents to never sweat the small stuff, and doing so came easily and naturally to her and her immediate family. It was so ingrained in her that she never got caught up in drama. My first impulse was to ask if her parents were looking to adopt.

What an amazing way to live! I wish that avoiding drama came naturally to me, but I had to learn the hard way how to deal with it.

A few years ago, I was wrapped up in the worst kind of mom drama around, and it honestly took me more than two years to recover. I had never had a falling-out with a friend before, but I did, and over something ridiculous. I felt wounded and defensive and hurt. We ended up not speaking to each other for a very long time, and the worst part was that the mutual friends we shared in a tight-knit group all stopped speaking to me as well. It was devastating. I didn't understand how these dear friends would just take the other side without ever talking to me about it. It was as if one day I existed and the next day I didn't. I had to walk into school with my head held high, be completely ignored, and pretend that I wasn't crying inside, day after day.

Before this happened, I would have never classified myself as an insecure person. What upset me the most was how it changed me in that way. For a long time, I second-guessed everything about my friendships. If someone didn't call me back right away I imagined the worst in my head. My ego was constantly going off, and I hated myself during that time.

As time went on and I felt less raw, I reflected on who I was at the time of that fight, what part I had to take responsibility for in the situation, and what lessons I learned. There were many. Time and space were the only things that allowed me to see how much I had grown and changed for the better since this happened.

Reconciliations have been made, long talks have taken place, and even though things will never go back to how they were, I am finally comfortable with all the women involved. I realize it took so long because I had to finally get comfortable with myself first.

If the same thing happened now, how would the "new and im-proved" me react? I can't imagine it would have gone so far. I would like to think that I would have picked up the phone, or driven over to my friends' houses to talk face-to-face about what happened and how we could resolve it. I like to think that I would have breathed through it all, and kept it in perspective. I would have asked the Universe to help me see the situation differently, and to acknowledge

my part in it. I would have asked for help, instead of feeling help-less.

I have also learned over the last few years that I'd rather have peace in my heart, mind, and soul than be right all the time. I don't always feel the need to prove my point because it doesn't matter if the other person agrees with me. As long as I am confident in my feelings that is all that matters, and they are, of course, entitled to their own.

I stood up to someone very close to me, and I am proud to say that it didn't freak me out nearly as much as it would have in the past.

I am very careful about whom I share my ideas with concerning angels, spirit, and reincarnation. There is an appropriate time and a place, and it is usually only if someone specifically asks me to share. I don't go around shouting my ideas from the rooftops, especially because they may seem unconventional, and I never want to make anyone uncomfortable. I also don't need to prove anything about my beliefs. They are mine, and they bring me comfort, joy, and peace, as I believe all feelings should.

This person in my life believed they were helping me by sending me articles about mediums that were fakes. I am not ignorant to the fact that there are many people who prey on those who so desperately want to believe. However, all of my experiences have felt extremely legitimate to me. I realize that this person felt that they had my best interests at heart, but I had had enough. I lovingly thanked them for their concern but also requested that they stop sending me these types of articles. For a while, I had just been deleting them, but I didn't even want the negative energy in my inbox. I thought that would be the end, and truth be told I was expecting an apology, but I got total backlash instead.

I was told that I must be so insecure in my beliefs that I couldn't stand to be exposed to the other side of the argument. This was the very first time in my life that I felt personally attacked in an argument, yet I felt completely calm at my center. I replied that, actually, the opposite was true—I felt so secure that I had no desire to prove anything. When you defend a position, it is typically because you want the other person to think you are right or agree with you. In this case, I felt entitled to my opinion, and I wasn't trying to sway anyone to believe what I believe. I didn't care about being right, so there wasn't anything to say. And with that, we agreed to disagree.

I cared much more about being at peace than being right. I was finally learning how to ride the waves.

Having had these experiences will only make me better able to guide my children as they inevitably navigate their own tough social predicaments. I know that they will go through similar experiences, so I can only hope that they will be better equipped to handle them than I was in the past.

20

Feel Your Feelings

"The truth will set you free, but first it will piss you off."
—GLORIA STEINEM

I spent most of my life suppressing anything that was hard to bear. My defense mechanism was pasting a giant smile on my face, and saying that I was "great!" Otherwise, life would have felt too hard, and I just wasn't ready to deal. This strategy worked for a long time and it got me through periods of my life that may have been very bleak otherwise, like counting out waitressing tips during my college years to see if I would make rent. For that I am grateful, but it got to the point where denying my feelings instead of acknowledging and accepting them was going to hold me back from growing as a person. There is only so far you can go with your head buried in the sand.

The further I traveled on my spiritual journey of self-discovery, the less choice I had about what was actually happening inside of me. I asked for guidance and support, and gave up having to feel like I was in control. I decided to sit back and enjoy the ride. I didn't have the chance to figure out if I was ready to finally face my feelings because they were steamrolling into my life no matter what. The Universe knew it was finally my time, even if I still had doubts.

I had meditations that didn't end up being meditations at all, but more of me crying in a ball on the floor of my closet, if you can even call it that. Howling, gasping, exploding, and touching places deep in my core that had never seen the light of day. I finally released any sort of control I had over my emotions and simply let them flood my being until I was all cried out. When there were no more tears, I would sit back up and breathe. When I guide meditations now, I often encourage people to allow their long deep breaths to be cleansing, nourishing breaths. I know how good it feels from experience. My breath soothed me and washed away all the sorrow, shame, and anger that I felt.

The only feelings that I had allowed myself to feel strongly up to this point in my life were the good ones. I had an immense and fierce love for my husband and kids. I actually saw a wonderful psychologist a few times after my first son was born because I needed help processing such an intense love. I had never felt emotion so strongly and it scared me a little bit.

Meditation was the only time that I had ever been still with myself. I had never heard silence before. Any downtime I ever had was spent on the phone, or reading, or listening to music. I had never been with my own thoughts, or witnessed what I was capable of feeling. Once these waves of emotion began washing over me I was cracked open in an entirely new way, and I never even thought of turning back. I began to understand that there were levels of self-awareness that, although new to me, were the key to my growth. I asked myself the really hard questions and found out how I REALLY felt inside. I was honest about my feelings for the very first time and faced all my demons and difficult memories head on.

I began to understand myself and know myself in a whole new way. I accepted the good, the bad, and the ugly. I didn't like everything I saw, but I examined my thoughts from different angles and accepted them. The real me emerged and I saw that I was kind and strong, and capable of fulfilling my dreams. As I healed myself, I knew it was my calling to shine my light and encourage others to do the same. Instead of making excuses, I heeded the call and began to live my purpose.

The only way that I have been able to sustain my growth and continue on this trajectory has been to question myself at each twist and turn. I have created a new normal where I check in with myself daily, asking the hard questions and loving myself no matter how my most authentic self-answers. I have learned that all feelings and emotions are okay, but every reaction to them isn't. I have learned not to react, but to respond. I do this by pausing when I feel triggered or stressed, and instead of saying or doing something that I may regret I take a moment to pause and evaluate the situation. I notice if I feel a "yum" or a "yuck" and move forward accordingly with a response that I feel good about.

I always try these days to surround myself with people who accept me for who I am. For so long I did and said what I thought others wanted me to instead of being myself. My husband has always been the one exception to that. He is the first man who I felt truly accepted me and loved me with all my idiosyncrasies and weird habits. I guess he is the first one to *really* know me. Before we met, I promised myself that I would never again pretend to be someone I am not. From the moment we met, Mark made me feel so comfortable, and

I knew he was a keeper! He loved me when I was a hot mess, and our bond has only strengthened the past sixteen years.

Hiding from my true self wasn't the answer, but timing was everything. I would have been a basket case if this happened a few years earlier. I believe in divine timing and trust it completely. Each one of us is just where we need to be right now. It is the right time and place for what is happening in our lives. The stars do align for each and every one of us when they are meant to. I have the utmost faith that the next phase of my growth will come just when I am ready for it. The questions may get even harder, but I will be up for answering them. It won't be a minute too late, or a minute too soon.

Do your emotions ever scare you to the point where you can't face them? I can promise you that there is another way—a different, and for most of us, a better way, whenever you are ready. And not a minute before.

Section 2

As-Needed Practices

Something I learned on my mindfulness journey is that there are periods of expansion and contraction. We can't do everything at once, and improvement takes time. There have been times I see myself catapulting forward at lightning speed, and there are others that I feel like I have stalled. I think sometimes we just need a chance to catch up to ourselves.

The times I feel at a spiritual standstill are the perfect times to call on the additional practices that I write about in this next section. Clearing clutter or making time to help others may be just what I need to clear my mental cobwebs and get out of my head and into the bigger, broader world around me. It always makes me feel better when I am caught up in my own sadness or worry to do something for others, or create a way to bring more love into my life and family.

Once we create habits and solidify a few everyday practices that feel good to start with, we can bring more awareness to what we need in times that feel challenging. I hope these serve you well!

21

Stress/Gratitude List

"The only power we have in our life is our attitude,
and that makes all the difference."

—MIMI IKONN

The kids are sick, practice ran late, you didn't get your workout in, and you realize that you left clothes in the washer for the entire day—sounds like a normal day, right? On days when it seems like everything is going wrong, we need to be reminded of how good we still have it.

I get stressed out occasionally just like everyone else, and I then feel guilty because I know there are people that have it way worse than I do. I have enough to eat, a warm and safe place to sleep, and my kids receive an education. However, it doesn't mean that my problems don't feel like problems as they are happening, nor that they aren't important in my life at the time.

It is important to keep them in perspective, though, and making a stress/gratitude list is a wonderful way to do this.

I originally saw this idea in a book by the amazing Michele Kambolis, used to help kids deal with stress. I became enamored by Michele after reading her book *Generation Stressed*, and my husband and I began working with her over the phone (she is in Canada) to get parenting advice and help with a few issues we were dealing with in terms of the boys. I cannot say enough good things about her. Every session was extremely valuable and informative. I am a huge proponent of "parenting sessions" in general. In these sessions with Michele, we got to ask anything we want about our kids, and how we were doing as parents. We typically kept notes of how we handled certain situations, and then asked Michele how we could have done it better in order to improve our parenting skills for the next situation. We have consulted a few people over the years, but working with Michele has given us the greatest results. I see my son transforming before my eyes, and it is a miracle to watch.

This is the way the list works:

Take out a piece of paper and draw a line down the middle, creating two columns. At the top of one side write "Stress," and at the top of the other write "Gratitude." Spend a few minutes writing down everything that is currently stressing you out on the Stress side of the page. Don't hold back because you don't have to show this list to anyone! They can be big things, little things, superficial things, whatever. You can even play a favorite song while you do this. Take as long as you need.

For every one thing that you are stressed about, you will write TWO things on the Gratitude side of the page. Again, these can be big things or small. When you are finished writing, you will see that even though you have things that you are stressed about, you have so much more to be grateful for.

What I love about this exercise is that it allows us to acknowledge the stress in our lives. We aren't ignoring it or feeling bad for having it. We are honoring our feelings of stress. At the same time, we have an amazing visual showing that no matter what, the good outweighs the bad. We always have more to be grateful for than worried about.

This can also be done on a smaller scale in the moment when needed. Instead of making a comprehensive list, you can simply conquer one worry at a time.

Take a small piece of paper, even a scrap, and write your worry on one side. Flip the paper over and write two things you are grateful for. Notice how good it feels to have more written on the gratitude side, and if doing so helped to alleviate your stress at all and gain a bit of perspective in the moment.

This exercise is also amazing to do with kids, and as Michele does, you can call it a worry/gratitude list. For older kids, this would be wonderful to do before a big test or finals.

22

Create Rituals

"Life isn't about finding yourself. Life is about creating yourself."
—GEORGE BERNARD SHAW

I love bringing more meaning to small acts with rituals. I already mentioned my morning ritual, but I have others as well. Some are all mine, and some I share with my family and friends.

Before I write a blog post, or during the writing of this book, I put peppermint oil behind my ears to perk me up, and then apply lip balm and cuticle oil. If I look down at my fingers and see dry cuticles I can easily get distracted picking them or wondering if I need a manicure, so it is really a preemptive move. Doing these things creates a definite time and space for my writing and makes it feel important and very intentional.

Before bed, I apply lip balm and cuticle oil again (I guess they're very dry), and I usually hop into bed with a book. These are additional opportunities for self-care which make *me* feel like a priority in my life. These small acts are done after I have taken care of dinner for my husband and kids, tucked the boys in, cleaned up downstairs, taken the dogs out one more time, written in my journal, and forced myself to wash my face even when I am exhausted. It signals to me at the end of a long day that I matter, and I can't forget to take care of myself. If I do, I will pay the price of cracked lips and scraggly cuticles!

I have a favorite store that I always pop in on when visiting my BFF in New York City. I can't imagine going to the city and not popping in. It's just part of what we do together. I also can't imagine visiting my twin sister and not walking up to the water tower near her house. It would just feel like something was missing if I didn't.

Maybe I like predictability, but I always take the same route on my runs, and on walks with my dogs. I am not completely anal about it, and if the mood strikes me to go a different way I honor that, it just rarely does. Turns seem to happen on their own, which leaves my attention free to soak up the beauty around me, or get inspired about a project.

We have created a few meaningful rituals as a family as well. On our boys' birthdays my husband and I decorate their rooms in a creative way for them to find when they wake up. It started with balloons and streamers in the doorway and graduated over the years to covering their whole bed with paper that they have to bust out of when they wake up. My husband and I are under the gun every year to think of something to outshine what we did the previous year. It is getting harder and harder, but the boys get so excited and actually start trying to guess what we will do a few days out, so we cannot disappoint them! It's a fun and bonding project for Mark and I to do together. We love it as much as they do.

I take the boys for Ice Cream Fridays as much as I can. These are simple outings to get ice cream after school, but giving it a title makes it feel special. After a long week, it is such a nice way to unwind with them and enjoy a treat.

Another fun thing we do is write on wish paper during the full moon. Wish paper is extremely thin paper that you write on, roll up into a cylinder, and light on fire. When it burns, it flies into the air and the ashes spread. It isn't dangerous, I promise! It is fun to watch and the kids and I enjoy writing our messages to the Universe about what we want to let go of, and what we hope to bring more of into the next month.

A dear friend has Sugar Cereal Saturday at her house. Since they eat a very healthy diet all week long, sugared cereal would never be allowed for breakfast, but every Saturday morning the rules don't apply and the kids can have whatever they want.

I was curious about what rituals families practiced, so I posted the question on my personal Facebook page, anxious to see what people shared. Here are a few replies that came in:

- We do a guided meditation as a family before bed.
- At dinner every night we would go around the table and share our highs and lows of the day. It was a great way to stay connected and to realize that life will always have ups and downs but your family is always there for you.
- Before bed, we name three things we are grateful for that day.
- We tuck our kids in and tell them how proud we are of them and why. Every single night.
- At dinner on Friday night, we whisper something in their ears that made us proud of them that week.

These rituals are simply ways to honor our relationships with each other and ourselves. I feel like I am making memories with my family when I keep these rituals going. However, I don't ever put too much pressure on myself about them. Some stick and some don't, and they don't have to last forever. The important thing is to enjoy them. Rituals should be adding special moments to your life, not stressing you out trying to make them happen (with the exception of the birthday ritual). If we have a commitment on a Friday and our ice cream date doesn't happen, we are all reminded of how important flexibility is in our lives. It is interesting to see which rituals each of my kids gravitate towards. I have said the same prayer every single night with my older son since he was two years old. It is the last thing we do together every night, and we have a special way of alternating words which has developed over the years. As much as he loves it, my younger son can take it or leave it. He cares much more about how his stuffed animals are lined up on his bed.

As I grow and transform, my rituals may change as well. It will be interesting to see what my pre-writing ritual is for my next book.

23

Acts of Kindness

"An act of kindness has the power to create miracles."
—DENISE LINN

There is never a wrong time to be kind. When I feel great I love nothing more than lifting the spirits of those around me to the same high vibration, and when I am in a crap mood, focusing on other people gets me out of my funk.

Some of my favorite acts of kindness include:

Giving compliments—Tell someone how nice their hair looks, or how yummy their food is, and watch them light up inside!

Leaving a comment on social media—Trust me, when someone posts on their blog, Instagram, or Facebook page, they want nothing more than to know that it resonated with someone. If you especially liked a post, let them know. You will make their day.

Reach out to an old friend—Is there someone you think about all the time and want to reconnect with? Don't wait another minute. Reach out. Chances are they have been thinking about you too.

Pay for the person in line behind you—It may just be a coffee or a bagel to you, but to them it imparts care and love. You also have the ability to impact all of the other people in line. Everyone around you may be inspired to also act with kindness.

Leave inspirational notes around town—Leave one with a tip on a table after a meal, under a windshield wiper on a car, or put one in with a bill that you mail. Whoever finds it will be so inspired. It only takes a moment to write "Have a nice day!"

Leave an extra big tip—I waitressed my way through college, and trust me, people in restaurants work hard! Leave an extra generous tip for someone who served you. It will really make his or her day.

Invite people into your home—Instead of always scheduling a coffee date at Starbucks, I invite people to my home and make a delicious hot drink for them. I love whipping out my milk steamer, and we usually curl up in my Zen den and talk an hour away. It is much more relaxing to be in a quiet, serene space.

Cook a meal for someone—I don't know if it is just a Houston thing, or southern hospitality in general, but everyone here is so generous with meals. When you have a baby, or surgery of any kind, people are lining up to help with meals. Family and friends have told me that this doesn't typically happen where they live, If it doesn't happen where you live, either, be a trendsetter!

Checking in—I do my best to remember if someone told me that they have an important doctor appointment or meeting coming up,

or something for their kids that they are worried about. I always do my best to follow up and see how it went. Sometimes I even put a reminder on my calendar because it is easy to forget when life gets busy.

Spontaneous texts—I don't always have something specific to say to someone, but I want them to know that I am thinking about them. It may feel weird to simply write "Hi," but why hold back? I send messages all the time that simply say, "Nothing much is going on, I just wanted you to know that I am thinking about you." I would love to get one of those!

The sky is the limit here. There is no way to screw up being nice, so go for it! If it would make you feel good, chances are someone else will like it too.

As important as it is to think of others, don't forget about yourself in the process. You are amazing and you should celebrate that whenever you get the chance! I encourage my coaching clients to do this all the time. If you achieved a goal, like meditating every day for a week, give yourself a treat. If you are having a rough day, don't wait for someone else to make you feel better; take control and do something nice for yourself. Some of my favorite ways to treat myself are:

- Buy an amazing dark chocolate bar and enjoy it piece by piece
- Treat myself to a mani/pedi
- I bust out the milk steamer for myself all the time and make one of my famous chai mistos. I am an addict!
- On nice days, I may blow off a task to spend more time outside enjoying nature.
- I buy a new lip gloss every three months to celebrate the change of season.

- I block time off for an extra yoga class or longer afternoon meditations when I know I need them.
- I'll curl up on the couch and read for fun or watch a show.

The more you perform acts of kindness for yourself and others, the more a natural part of your routine they become. Start with a goal of one a week for someone else and yourself and take it from there.

24

Make a Wish List

"Believe you can and you're halfway there."
—THEODORE ROOSEVELT

As the years whiz by, it hits me that if I don't start achieving some lifelong goals that I have set for myself, I just may miss my chance. Some days I feel like I have no clue where the past ten years have gone, and I don't want to let ten more pass me by in a blur without seeing the big picture.

Being a book enthusiast, I have dreamed for years of writing my own. I even started writing one about eight years ago, but never finished. The main character was based on me, and when I reread what I wrote, I decided I didn't like the main character at all (maybe that should have been my first clue that I had some serious internal work and soul searching to do). It took me years to figure out what kind of book I wanted to write, but when I knew I knew, and here we are. I had so much in my heart that I wanted to share with other moms, and I knew that if I didn't just sit down and write, I would always regret it. I didn't want to think about "what if?" anymore.

Is there something that you have been wanting to do for a long time? It could be taking up yoga, giving up sugar, taking ballroom dance lessons, driving a race car, scuba diving, or having a three-some—the sky is the limit!

I made a list of everything I wanted to accomplish in the next few years and it had things on it like:

- Write a bestselling book
- Get rid of the muffin top I have had since my kids were born
- Speak to a large audience
- Balance in crow position in yoga class

The items on the list can certainly change as you do. These have been big ones for me for a while, and before it was too late, I got going on one. That is why you are reading this book. Writing it was something I could talk about forever, or a goal that I could work toward day by day until I accomplished it. It also seemed a lot less daunting than dealing with the muffin top!

I knew it wasn't possible to deal with everything on my list at one time, so I decided to start with one, and it just so happened to be the one that would cause me the most regret if I didn't do it.

If you made a list, what is the first thing that you would tackle? Whatever that thing is, you should do it. The fact that you are reading this book just goes to show that anything is possible!

25

Volunteer

"The best way to find yourself is to lose yourself in the service of others."
—GANDHI

No matter how long my to-do list is, I wake up excited on the days I am volunteering. In part 11, I mentioned that it took a while for me to find the perfect volunteer fit, but now that I have, I am crazy about what I do to serve others.

Volunteering at a place where I didn't know anyone when I got there opened me up to a whole new group of wonderful friends that I would have never met. I leave my comfortable bubble for four hours a month, and I am not Mark's wife, or Adam and Dylan's mom, I am simply Ali. I find immense joy in making someone else's life better, putting a smile on their faces, and building their confidence. I can put everything aside that is going on in my life to focus on someone who needs me. I try to be a good person all the time, but, in those four hours a month, I am my very best self. Although I am giving my time, I receive so much in return. I am given the gift of being in the moment because anything going on in my life falls away.

I encourage you to make volunteering a priority in your life, whether it be for one hour a week, one hour a month, or one time a year. Organizations need extra help during the holidays, and that is a wonderful time to help out.

We now make holiday volunteering a family affair. My husband had been involved in Elves and More for a few years on his own. He helped build bicycles to be given out to deserving kids before Christmas, and always talked about how incredible it was to see thousands of bikes built by volunteers lined up to be donated.

As soon as our kids were old enough, we started going as a family to build the bikes, and then a few days later we would go to the schools to help give them out to the kids. I have never been more proud of my boys. They worked so hard and loved every minute of it. Seeing them help kids pick out their dream bike also gave them the opportunity to realize that it isn't about them all the time.

A few years ago, I decided that there was nothing more I wanted to do on my birthday than volunteer. I didn't want a party, and I didn't even want lunch out with friends. All I wanted to do was to help other people. It was an urge that I had, and every time I thought about how nice it was going to be I started to cry. Hormones, maybe? I was very emotional about it all. I asked some close family members and dear friends to come with me, and we all brought our kids as sous chefs to cook a meal for cancer patients at a residential facility run by volunteers. As my birthday gift, my cousins bought the groceries we needed to prepare the food, and we spent a few precious hours, moms and kids, cooking delicious homemade meals filled with love and care. We chopped, rolled out dough, and laughed. It was so much fun—and, of course, I was an emotional mess that day, too. Tears rolled down my cheeks as I thanked everyone for making it the most special birthday of my life. I will 100 percent continue to volunteer on my birthday, and have done so ever since.

Just like money, time is currency too. We may not all be in the position to give lots and lots of money away, even though in our hearts we would love to, so we need to give what we can. We need to find our middle. We may have more time, or we may have more money, and both make a huge difference to a needy organization. There is no way you can go wrong, as long as you do something.

Life is busy, but realistically we can all find a little pocket of time to help others. By doing so we are modeling for our kids how important it is to help others in need no matter what is going on in our own lives, as well as creating special memories. Here are some great ways to volunteer as a family:

- Volunteer at an animal shelter cleaning cages and giving the animals some much-needed attention.
- Make brown-bag lunches for a homeless shelter to give out. My kids love doing this!
- Make cards for adults or kids in the hospital.
- Bake cookies, or cook a meal for a person in your neighborhood that is sick.
- Drop off baked goods to the local fire station or police station.
- Adopt a family during the holidays and provide gifts and a meal that will make their holiday dreams come true.

Even if what you are doing feels insignificant to you, I promise you are making a huge difference in someone else's life. You will feel pretty amazing too. Talk about a win-win.

26

Clean UP!

"Clutter is nothing more than postponed decisions."
—BARBARA HEMPHILL

I have no separation between my roles as wife, mom, and entrepreneur. My to-do list is often comprised of writing a new script for a class, preparing a webinar, picking up deodorant for my husband, and ordering a braided belt for my fourth grader. I also work out of my home, which means that my office is also the mudroom. I love that I am home so much and don't have to commute to work, but it can be difficult to keep my life organized inside a 5 × 10 room.

I used to be a total Type-A, self-proclaimed neat freak. Being über-organized is one of the best qualities I got from my dad, and I am the only one of four siblings that inherited it. I am the sister that visits, organizes the fridge, and cleans off your kitchen counters.

Somewhere along the road of raising kids I realized that I was always buzzing around like a busy bee, doing dishes because I couldn't stand to have them in the sink, running clothes up to the laundry room so they wouldn't be laying around, and straightening the book cabinet so it was nice and neat when you opened the door, instead of actually reading those books with my kids . . . So, I eased up. I played games on the floor and did dishes later. I let stacks accumulate in my office, and I occasionally had to take uniform pants out of the laundry for a second wearing. I was prioritizing time with my kids, which felt very right in my heart, but something was nudging me in the gut.

I eased up until I couldn't stand to even sit in my office anymore. I had piles and stacks, unorganized files, and jumbles of cords so big that when I grabbed them with two hands to organize, it was so overwhelming that I just decided to shove them back on the shelf. Now, most of this mess was contained to my office, which I made the excuse of being my "messy room." I was okay with this exception as long as the rest of my house was neat, or at least looked neat when company showed up. I had a few cabinets and drawers that were a total wreck but nobody could see them, which made it okay (sort of).

Both the New Year starting, and being really ready to take my business to a new level in 2015, made me say ENOUGH, and I hired a professional organizer to help me whip my house, and mainly my office, into shape. I felt overwhelmed by the project but didn't want that to stand in the way of getting it done.

We had a consultation so I could show her all of the areas I wanted to work on, and within minutes I was bawling to this poor woman. I was overcome with emotion and started spilling my guts to someone I had never even met before.

What came pouring out is how I found it hard to balance being present with my kids while keeping up the house and running a growing business. I am running a business I love and adore, that fuels me beyond belief, out of a tiny office strewn with shoes and backpacks.

I write next to a huge pile of papers, and there is nothing that feels productive or abundant about that. It was obvious that I needed to find more balance in my space, and that things feeling organized and neat was crucial so that I could focus on my family and my work. I needed to clean up areas of my life that were out of control so that I could be successful and present in the really important ones.

This project facilitated self-awareness about issues I didn't even realize I had. I now consider taking care of my spaces to be self-care because an organized environment helps me stay clear and open to creativity, new ideas, and the flow of life. An organized space keeps me in the present moment and allows me to focus on one thing at a time, whether it be my family, my work, or myself.

Just like I teach others to do, I exhaled all the stress I felt associated with this project and inhaled the joy in knowing I was ready to tackle it. Together we made a game plan and determined what I needed to do on my own, prep-wise. I certainly didn't need the organizer to sit with me at an hourly rate to watch me clean out papers and old markers. I spent a few days over the holidays cleaning out drawers and cabinets until my husband asked me if I was pregnant and nesting again.

Then my organizer came back, and we spent four hours together in my home and another hour buying out the Container Store. I swear, I could spend all day in there! I also had one trip to OfficeMax which was less overwhelming and a little more affordable.

I now have a place for everything, and I can actually see my desk. When I sit in my office, I feel inspired instead of distracted. We also organized all my kids' "stuff" in the kitchen so that they know where to find everything, and more importantly, put everything away. I am hoping this fosters more independence in the boys and helps me to expect it from them.

When I gazed at the finished product my first thought was, "What took me so long?" I very well could have suffered through another year surrounded by my piles and crap, but I am so glad that I bit the bullet and got started. This is very much a metaphor for life. We can eat healthy next year, write that book in a month, or learn to meditate one day. But if we put off what we are seeking, what are we missing out on now? Obviously, it disturbed something inside of me to be surrounded by chaos. I didn't want to bring that energy into one more day, month, or year than I needed to.

What project can you tackle that will bring more calm, presence, and peace to your life? How can you prioritize your needs and desires by admitting what you need from your space and relationships? Can you make a plan to facilitate the change? I know you can. Take a moment and tell yourself what you are going to clear in your space/relationships/life to make room for what you want. Join me, because I still have several more rooms to go!

27

Get Inspired

"Go the extra mile. It's never crowded."
—UNKNOWN

When I put my iPod on and get moving on a clear, sunny day, everything else disappears. It's my favorite time to think, focus on myself, and soak up inspiration from the Universe. It never ceases to amaze me how many ideas I get when I am running outside.

Running has become a true passion, even though it was something I never even thought about until I was in my 30s. I wish I had known how much I loved it sooner. I might have actually been good at a sport growing up!

After the birth of my second child, I decided to run a half marathon with my neighbor. I had never run more than a mile before, but I knew it would be a feasible way to get my body back, and it turned out to be a wonderful experience for me. I came to enjoy many aspects of running, most importantly that I could leave my house and

be done in 30 minutes knowing that I had a great workout without having to leave the kids for too long.

Three months after the half marathon, I had a suspicious mole removed. Skin cancer didn't run in my family, and I truly didn't think too much of it. A week later I received a call from my dermatologist telling me that the mole was melanoma, but it wasn't life threatening "this time," since they caught it early. Less than a week later, I kissed my husband and two young sons goodbye as I was wheeled into surgery to have any excess cells removed and be cleared of cancer. The experience was a huge shock to me, scary as anything, and tremendously eye-opening. We all know that health is everything, yet sometimes it takes an unfortunate situation such as this one to bring focus to what is really important. I was so thankful that the cancer was caught early, but I was still angry at my seemingly healthy body.

My twin sister called shortly after my surgery to ask me if I would run the Philadelphia marathon with her; I was overcome with a mixture of fear and excitement. I called my husband to make sure he was on board, considering he would be holding down the fort while I trained, and Mark really pushed me to go for it. I will always be grateful for that push. I was excited to do something positive with my body and feel confident in my health again. The marathon was a huge success—truly one of the most extraordinary experiences of my life. I often say it was the fourth best day I ever had, after my wedding and the birth of each of my children. I had a smile on my face the entire way, in complete awe of what I had trained my body and mind to accomplish, for a marathon really is mind over matter. I felt incredibly happy and healthy, and it was a way for me to put my melanoma scare behind me.

I ran the Houston marathon with my twin sister the following year, and that was the official end of my long distance running career.

It was so much harder on my body the second time, and I decided that I would rather enjoy running three miles a few times a week for the next twenty years than hurt myself attempting long distances again. Even though on beautiful days I wish I could run for hours, it feels good to honor my body and truly listen to its signals. Instead of focusing on a limitation, I focus on the gift of those three glorious miles.

When I am trying to think of an idea for my writing, or what to do for an upcoming class, or how to handle a problem with my kids, or how to say "no" to something nicely, the first thing I do is lace up my sneakers and hit the pavement for thirty minutes. It is incredible what I receive, and I know that I can count on my runs to help clear my head and boost my creativity. I often visualize the amazing things I will accomplish while on my runs, and I can actually feel the sensations of being on a stage giving a talk, or leading a group, or whatever else I am hoping will come to fruition. I plan conversations in my head and write emails to people that I am frustrated with. I may never send them, but even thinking about what I would say makes me feel better.

Where do you feel your most inspired and creative? It is important to know so you have a game plan when you need a little boost. What clears your head and gets those creative juices flowing?

For me, it's running outside, but everyone has a different thing that calls to them. Maybe your time is while you cook, take a bath, or walk your dogs. It could be talking to a dear friend, writing in your journal, or praying. It is important to make whatever it is a regular part of your routine so that you don't feel blocked and weighed down. Let inspiration seep into you regularly.

28

Be Intentional with Your Attention

"Attention is love."

—SARAH McLEAN

I don't believe in coincidences, but I do believe in the synchronicity of the Universe; we can see signs of this if we are open to looking. When synchronicities happen in my daily life they feel like treasured gifts bestowed upon me, as if the Universe is trying to show me that it has my back. Because I am always on the lookout, I am able to notice them all the time and appreciate them fully. I always offer a short, silent prayer of thanks to the heavens when they occur because honestly, they just plain make me feel good.

I read a passage in *A Course in Miracles* early one morning after my meditation that really spoke to me. It said, "Peace, joy, and love abide in me." What a beautiful message, and what an amazing outlook to have as you move through life. So many people feel like the deck is constantly stacked against them, and this is the total opposite perspective. If you are filled with peace, joy, and love, anything seems possible.

About two hours later I was driving my kids to school, and somehow we began talking about doing good deeds. I had one of those "aha!" moments and I decided to use my lesson from *ACIM* that morning and convey the beautiful message to my children.

I told them, "You know guys, doing nice things for others comes naturally to you because you are filled with peace, love, and light. We all have a spark of God's goodness in us, and when we do nice things for others our spark grows brighter." My nine-year-old replied, "Yes, Mom, but we all have hatred in us too." Adam always enjoys highlighting the other side of whatever I am saying, which creates an environment for some pretty great conversations.

I explained to him that yes, we all do have a bit of hatred in us as well. It is normal to be filled with positive and negative feelings, but it is up to us to decide where to put our attention. We always have a choice. If we put our attention on the good stuff, like love and joy, that is what grows in our lives. If we put our attention on negativity, that is what will grow. We have the power to be intentional with our attention. We decide which emotions to focus on so that they can have more space in our thoughts and lives.

It is important to surround ourselves with people who are focused on the same things we are. If you have a group of friends or family members who focus on gossip and negativity all the time, it is easy to fall into the trap of joining into the judgment and complaining because you are surrounded by it. We need to be brutally honest with ourselves and decide who and what situations feel right to us. Who gives us the "yums" and what situations give us the "yucks." I am not advocating turning your back on friends or family, but sometimes a little distance is necessary for growth. As you raise your vibrations with positivity, not everyone will come along for the ride. The ebb and flow of relationships is part of life, and we can see it as good or bad, depending on where we put our attention. I look at it as a natural part of life and my personal evolution. The more in touch with my intuition I get, the more honest I can be with myself as to who and what feels good. This has happened in many areas of my life.

There are people in my life I am closer to now, and others I have drifted from. Honestly, this part was really hard for me, and still is at times. It is a combination of time and feelings. Now that I am building a business and working, I don't have as much time for lunches and coffees and hours on the phone. I have definitely pulled back socially to concentrate on fulfilling my purpose. I am still social, but a whole lot less. Right now, the boys really want me to tuck them in, and that isn't going to last forever, so I don't want to miss too many opportunities to savor their snuggles. It's when our best conversations happen, so I have gotten pickier as to what I am missing it for.

My marriage needs attention as well. Mark is my best friend and partner, but I don't want to ever take that for granted. It is so easy to put all my energy into the kids until all of a sudden I realize that we haven't had a real conversation about something else in a few days. I try to be careful about that, but it is amazing how the days fly, and by nighttime we are so tired.

And, last but not least, is ME. I need attention, too. I cannot allow myself to get depleted or I won't be able to care for anyone. The older I get, the more that time alone really fuels me. I feel like I am on a see-saw and I need to try to find the right balance of caring for others and myself if I ever want it to level out.

Our attention can easily get pulled in so many directions, but we need to have the courage and self-respect to draw boundaries and place our precious attention in the places that honor who we are and what is important to us.

It can be hard to turn down a volunteer opportunity, but if your child is having a hard time in school and needs extra homework help, you may have to. If you want to make family meal times a priority, then another after-school activity may have to wait until next semester. If another couple asks for plans but you haven't had a date with your husband in weeks, a date may take precedence. It is all about balance, and finding what works for you and your family.

The need for attention in different areas may shift, and we should be prepared to be flexible. Being honest with ourselves and listening to our intuition are the only real tools we need to be successful in the realm. The desire to put our energy, focus, and attention on the good stuff will make it easier for the good stuff to find us. I believe this with 100 percent certainty.

29

Hand It Off to the Universe

"If you are brave enough to say goodbye,
life will reward you with a new hello."
—PAULO COEHLO

No matter how much progress I make, and how much I learn and grow, sometimes I still don't have a clue of what to do. I hope I am not the only one! When I am stuck on how to deal with a situation or person, and the usual things like getting out of my head and into my body aren't working, I simply need to hand it over to the Universe.

I have said it before, and I'll say it again: The Universe has our backs. Believing this can change everything.

When I am fresh out of ideas for how to handle something in my personal or business life, I ask for guidance. This may seem a little unconventional, but don't turn the page yet because this stuff works and it is awesome!

I have a special box that I put notes to the Universe in. I call it my Worry Box. I write notes asking for guidance whenever I need help or want to manifest something in my life. I simply write something like:

I am confused about _____. I know there is another way to see this situation. Please show me what I need to know. Please guide me in the right direction so I can see things clearly. I accept any part I have played in making this hard and I release any negative feelings toward the situation. I am grateful for any insight concerning _____ and I will be open to any signs or feelings that come. Thank you.

I fold up the note, put it in the box, and go about my day. There has never been an immediate action, like a bolt of lightning striking and, all of a sudden, I know what to do. However, usually within two or three days I will notice a shift, and a feeling or inner knowing about how to proceed. Answers have come to me while I am stopped at a traffic light, while I am on a walk, or while brushing my teeth. A complete calm comes over me and I feel totally secure in how I am to move forward.

This has also become an amazing exercise in patience for me. I have always been all about immediate action and wanting to cross things off my list, but now I have transitioned into someone who is willing to wait for the right answer.

It is a comforting feeling to know that I don't have to go at it alone. Of course, I have my husband, friends, and family who are always there for me to talk things out with, but this just feels different because I am waiting until I have an overwhelming feeling of knowing what is right for me. It isn't based on anyone else's vision or opinion, but what is the truth for me. The Universe has my back, and it has yours too.

30

Let the Good Times Roll

"Sisters are like fat thighs . . . they stick together."
—UNKNOWN

It makes me sad sometimes that it is so much easier to remember the lousy parts of growing up than the good ones. When I think about growing up, the hardship is what sticks out, but there were good times too.

My kids love hearing stories about when Mark and I were young, and I often have trouble racking my brain for a good one. Before all hell broke loose when I was eleven, there were fun and special times. I remember things like listening to the Thompson Twins in my oldest sister's car, her taking me to see the Jackson 5, INXS, and *Dirty Dancing*. I remember riding bikes for hours with my twin sister, copying each other's homework, and making up dance routines with our best friend to "Walk Like an Egyptian." We wore poodle skirts and performed in the fifth-grade talent show to "Lollipop" even though neither one of us could dance. (We had another friend who carried the routine, thank goodness.) My middle sister was the coolest person on earth to me. I worshiped her. She was pretty hard on my twin and me, but we were happy to sit in her doorway to watch her and her friends when we weren't allowed in her room. When she went out, I would race to her room to snoop and look at every single item she owned with awe, like each one was a precious jewel.

My dad used to take us to an old-school barber shop downtown when he got his hair cut, and then out for special lunches. My mom allowed me to lay my head on her lap when she drove and she would tickle my back. (Obviously, this was before wearing a seatbelt was expected.) We had family dinners every single weeknight, and, for dessert, we always had "luscious fruit." We still tease my mom about that!

It is amazing that the four of us girls all remember different things. We are trying to do more reminiscing when we are all together because once we get going it is so much fun. Susan hates when we remind her of how she used to rent us her clothing growing up. Until my parents found out, she capitalized on my twin and me with a price list in her closet of what we had to pay to wear her clothes. We remind Steph about all the times she wanted to eat dinner under the table and pretend she was a dog, and they love to tease me about how I used to stomp my feet obsessively when I got mad. Old habits die hard; it took me a while to stop, and even as an adult I have stomped occasionally. Fortunately though, not in the past couple of years!

I find it so grounding to share these stories and focus on the good times we shared growing up. They are a part of me, and the more we reminisce, the more I remember. It is also an important reminder to take the time to create memories as a family, and to realize that they don't have to be grand experiences. It is in the everyday that the treasures lay. The gems are the stories we tell about everyday life, and that is why living in the present moment is so important. I want to enjoy every small moment spent with my little family.

It's funny that you think you will never forget anything about your kids. Somehow many of the details have blurred, and I can't remember exactly how old each one was when they said their first word and got their first tooth. As each event happened, it felt so important that I thought I'd never forget a single detail, but I did. The lesson is to write it down, or not worry about it and just enjoy each event as it occurs.

My kids are always asking me to photograph and video them doing everything. I do take pictures and video at some big events, but I have explained to them that I want to be in the moment with them, enjoying what they do, and not behind a camera all the time. It is a different experience to be truly present and enjoying something versus worrying about getting a good shot. I have become more discerning about when to bust out my camera—unless something is likely to be a defining moment that absolutely needs to be documented, I simply try to stay in the present moment and enjoy life as it happens.

31

Be Flexible

"If you don't like how things are, change it! You're not a tree."
—JIM ROHN

During the course of this journey of personal growth, I have learned to be flexible with myself. I have tried techniques that I am not sharing in this book because although they are extremely valuable, and have changed the lives of many, they just didn't stick for me.

Part of honoring your journey is trying lots of different things and learning to admit what works for you, and what doesn't. Some things I tried for a while but didn't stay consistent with, like practicing kundalini yoga in the early mornings before my seated meditation Even though I wanted more time to practice, I felt rushed, and it was just too much for me. Now doing kundalini is more of an "as needed" practice or an extra treat in my day.

One quality I shed along the way was the need to compare myself to others. In years past I may have been embarrassed to admit if a self-help technique that someone loved didn't work for me. I would

have wondered if something was fundamentally wrong with me. A slew of insecurities would have come forth, and I may have stumbled over my words and questioned my judgment.

These days I am more into individuality and testing the waters. I am open-minded and interested in everything related to spirituality, yet not everything is a fit for me. I have to be honest with myself and listen to my intuition about where to focus my attention. This skill is tested often as I am bombarded with information and offers about the amazing programs and retreats being offered. In a perfect world, I would attend them all, but I am not in a place to do that right now. I have to pick and choose very carefully and be confident in the fact that timing is everything. I will say yes to something when I am meant to be there, or I need to learn from that program, and not a moment sooner. I try not to think of it as missing out on an opportunity, but more as though I am letting divine timing take over.

Flexibility can be hard to master, but it is such a gift. We don't have to pretend to have all the answers right this minute. We can turn life into a puzzle and freak out if we don't have all of the pieces put together by a certain deadline that we set, or we can enjoy the process more by calmly searching through the pile till we find the right piece.

I would say that this has been one of the hardest concepts for me to master, but my life is so much more joyful without all that self-inflicted pressure to make everything work. Some things stick and some don't, but they all make life more interesting.

Section 3

Attitude Adjustments

The more we practice our mindfulness tools, the more natural it becomes to use them, and the more they help us in overwhelming and stressful times. However, if your life is anything like mine, situations will inevitably occur that require a little extra attention above the norm. For me, they often have to do with the way I see certain situations or relationships, and ultimately myself. This is where my attitude adjustments come into play.

Attitude adjustments happen when I recognize a thought pattern or behavior in myself that needs a little upgrade.

While on a journey to live a more mindful life, not everything we begin to notice about ourselves is awesome. Not everything makes us feel proud, and some of it can be downright shocking! I remember thinking on more than one occasion, *holy cow, I have more work to do than I thought!* I still do at times today.

In order to grow, we must be willing to be uncomfortable. We must be willing to embrace all our thoughts and emotions so we can

make sense of them, and work through them to become the best version of ourselves.

This is the section of the book where I get the most vulnerable. I talk about some big-time issues that I had to work through. They were tough. They were painful. But I am sick of feeling ashamed—these situations don't define me. What I learned from them, and the fact that I moved forward in a better way, does.

Nobody has cornered the market on hardship. Everyone has pain in their life, it's just that the manifestation is different.

I had to get over feeling embarrassed of my past, and simply embrace that it is my story. Sharing my truth has helped me connect to more people, and impact their lives so they don't feel as alone.

I don't hide the parts of myself that aren't shiny and pretty like I used to. Pretending everything was perfect didn't serve me; it actually stunted my growth. Being honest feels great. So, here it goes!

32

Different Doesn't Mean Bad

"Never regret. If it's good, it's wonderful. If it's bad, it's experience."
—VICTORIA HOLT

Before I learned to live in the flow, I always had an idea in my mind of how things should be. If things didn't happen the way I wanted them to I would get stressed, stressed, and more stressed—it was a wasteful way to live. I brought so much unnecessary drama into my life and wasted so much energy focusing on the wrong things. I was so uptight and I was constantly disappointed by people.

I was so insecure that my ego, the part of our minds that focuses on lack, judgment, and insecurity, had free reign over my brain most days. I took everything personally and made a lot of assumptions. If someone canceled plans on me, instead of understanding that life gets in the way, my mind would go to a very dark place and create a situation in my head where that person didn't care about me or prioritize our friendship at all.

Through meditation, I was able to gain much better control of my emotions. I learned how to deal with situations that triggered me and make better choices for myself. I also learned to loosen the reins a bit. Things happen for a reason. Different doesn't mean bad, and sometimes a cosmic redirection is needed in order to create space for something different—maybe even better. If you look hard enough, there is usually a lesson of some kind tucked away in every stressful situation.

A perfect example is when I started my online group coaching program. Looking back, I had a desperate energy around it. I was in the middle of a few other big projects and I kind of just threw it out there without putting forth the right energy and intention around it. I honestly just expected people to sign up, but you know what? They didn't.

At first, I was really disappointed and embarrassed, but I realized that the Universal lesson of timing was at play here. I pulled back and regrouped. I waited until the timing was right. I rewrote my marketing materials so that my intention of serving to the best of my ability could be felt. Positive energy oozed out of my posts, and I handed the issue of registrationoff to the Universe. I told myself that the right people would be attracted to this program, and I was right.

The right people did sign up. The ones that needed this program came, and now it is one of my absolute favorite things I do. I look forward to the bi-monthly calls and am buzzed with high vibes when they end. Everyone in the program is learning and expanding in amazing ways, and I am honored to be a part of their journey.

This is a prime example of how when we push too hard nothing happens, but when we open up our lives, the miraculous has a chance to come forward.

These days, if someone cancels on me, I feel like the Universe opened up space and time to run an errand, write a bit, or take an extra walk. I don't automatically jump to that place of negativity like I used to so easily. It's all about perspective. This is one of the most meaningful shifts that I have seen in my life, and it feels wonderful to jump to the positive instead of the negative. The book *The Four Agreements* was on my reading list in Section 7, and for the purpose of letting go of assumptions and not taking things personally I can't recommend it enough. It is actually required reading for all my private coaching clients. I am begging you to order it today!

33

Don't Be Afraid of the Journey

"You don't always need a plan. Sometimes you need to breathe, trust, let go, and see what happens."

—MANDY HALE

I was talking to a dear friend about this very topic because she was having a very difficult time figuring out how she wanted to re-enter the workforce when her youngest started kindergarten. She had a few options but couldn't figure out what felt exactly right, and she was making herself nuts. I told her that she needed to take some of the pressure off herself and realize that she didn't have to commit to something for the rest of her life. She could get a job, and if after a while it didn't seem like a fit, or she wanted to do something else, she could. I assured her that she never had to be embarrassed to admit that she wanted to try something new.

I have always been about the journey, not the destination.

I have held many jobs in different fields. I was always looking for the one that lit me up inside, and it wasn't until I started teaching meditation that I finally felt that way. I wake up every single morning excited about what lies ahead, and I truly feel that every job I have had up until this one prepared me in some way to reach my full potential.

When I graduated college, I worked in corporate America planning events and helping to run our company's volunteer program. It was an amazing job that I felt grateful to have, but after about three years the stress of event planning got to me, and I knew it was time to move on.

I decided to leave the corporate sector, and I became the development director at a private school. I learned that development was not for me because I absolutely hated asking people for money, which was a huge part of the job. What I did find out is that I loved the atmosphere of a school, so, after two years in development, I decided to become a teacher.

I got my teaching certificate and started teaching kindergarten. The fact that I was allowed to be alone with 24 five-year-olds, day in and day out, speaks volumes of what is wrong with our education system. I had no clue what I was doing. I loved the kids, but I was a decent teacher at best. I got pregnant during my second year and decided to stay at home with my son (thank goodness for everyone, especially the kindergartners).

Being a mom was the first thing that felt totally right, and two years after Adam was born, Dylan came along. My heart somehow expanded as every mom promises it will, and I was head over heels in love with both my boys. My days were filled with playing at the water table, reading stories, and making homemade meatballs with veggies hidden in them. I wouldn't trade these years for anything, but as the kids got a little older and started preschool I began to crave a way to find more fulfillment in the hours when I was alone. I was filling my mornings with going to the gym and meeting friends for coffee, but I had too much downtime that I felt could be put to use in better ways.

I wanted to contribute financially to our family in some way, so I piggy-backed off my teaching certificate and got certified as a reading specialist. The hours were perfect, but I dreaded going to tutor each and every day. Obviously, it wasn't a good fit.

Social media and blogs had really grown by then, so I decided to try my hand at writing. For five minutes I had a blog called Ali's Obsessions. You might not realize this, but I am a sharer. If I like something I tell everyone about it. I am passionate about sharing things I love, whether it be a beauty product or a recipe. So, for Ali's Obsessions, I basically wrote blog posts about things I loved. I really enjoyed it, and I liked being online, but I wanted to take it one step further. I wanted to tackle a subject with a little more depth, and I wanted to be of even more service to others.

After having two kids, my relationship with my mother-in-law began to blossom. I needed her help in a major way; my own mom lived halfway across the country, and my mother-in-law was always generous with her time watching the kids. It wasn't that our relationship before that was bad, but we weren't particularly close, and I can honestly say that it was all me. I often felt resentful of unsolicited advice concerning my children and pretty much shut down during most conversations with her. I can admit now that it took me needing her help, and knowing that I had to be nicer if I wanted her to help me, for me to let her in more. My mother-in-law is a really good person, and by keeping her at a distance I was only hurting myself.

It was obvious from talking to all my friends that every daughter-in-law felt that they were navigating choppy waters when it came to their in-laws. I had seen how my relationship with mine developed over the years and I thought I could help others through their own difficult times. I felt that there had to be a way to bring young women together to bond and support one another in bettering the daughter-in-law/mother-in-law relationship.

I started a website called Daughter-in-Law Diaries to help women everywhere tackle and improve their relationship with their in-laws. The best part was that I had two amazing therapists who would answer questions that readers wrote in; they gave incredible advice and helped solve some pretty tough dilemmas for some pretty desperate people. I loved that we were helping people, but the website never really took off, and after two years I shut it down so I could pursue other passions.

About here is where my love for meditation grew, and when I felt with my whole heart that my purpose was to inspire, teach, and guide others to bring meditation and mindfulness into their lives in a really relatable way. I firmly believe that my business began to take off because of everything I learned from the previous jobs I had. I knew that I wanted to serve, help, and inspire, and each job I held in the past, even though it wasn't a perfect fit, taught me something I brought into what I am doing now. I grew as a person and a professional from each job I had, and learned more about myself and what I wanted with each one. If I hadn't had a website before, building one for my teaching practice would have been completely overwhelming. If I hadn't commanded a classroom in the past, I may not be as confident as a presenter and teacher now. Each experience builds on the last as our skill set develops and we find our true passion.

There were times I felt like a complete flake. Why couldn't I figure out what I wanted to be when I grew up? I felt embarrassed to say that I was trying something else, as if anyone really cared. They didn't. I came to the realization that nobody, with the exception of

my husband, really cared what I was up to. My family and friends wanted me to be happy, period. If it took trying career after career to do that, so be it.

Maybe it is because I have finally found "it" that I can say this, but I am proud that I had the confidence to keep trying, and that I never settled for something that didn't feel right just to prove that I could stick it out.

I love what I do. Guiding and inspiring others to transform their lives from the inside out is an honor and privilege. I hope that I am doing this forever, but I will always be open to the journey. Who knows where my teaching, coaching, writing, and motivational speaking will lead.

If you are looking for permission to try something new in your life, I am giving it to you. If I can do it, you can too. Go after what you truly want, and keep in mind that sometimes we don't know what that is right away. Enjoy the process of finding out, with an open mind and an open heart.

34

Laugh at Yourself

"If you are always trying to be normal you will never know how amazing you can be."

—MAYA ANGELOU

This is a biggie! Life is no fun if we take it seriously all the time. As long as nobody gets seriously injured, we have to learn to laugh at the crazy experiences along the way.

I am constantly doing and saying stupid and embarrassing things, especially when I get nervous. The worst is that I always seem to say something ridiculous at doctors' appointments and they always look at my like I have two heads. I get the worst nervous giggles at the gynecologist, which is so awkward! Sometimes I wish I was just a nice, quiet girl, but that isn't how I was built.

I got a lot of practice at laughing at myself in high school when it came to my first car.

When I was sixteen, I desperately wanted my own form of transportation, mostly so I didn't have to beg for rides to my part-time

job. I scraped together $1,000 that I saved from working, and was enough for basic car insurance, and bought a dilapidated, stick shift station wagon. I grew up in a very affluent suburb of Philadelphia, and my high school parking lot was filled with BMWs, brand new Jeeps, and of course a plethora of Toyota Celicas. I dreamed of driving that car—it was the epitome of cool.

My second day driving I got into a horrible accident. I turned left at a light without waiting for the people in the other direction to go straight because I was concentrating so hard on not stalling, and dealing with the stick shift, that when I saw green I just went. The whole side of my car got smashed in, which of course my basic insurance didn't cover. For two years I drove a car with a bashed-in side, and, instead of a window, I had a piece of Plexiglas duct-taped to the door. Every week or so the duct tape would have to be replaced, and now that I think about how much money I spent on duct tape over two years, I may have been able to fix the door. The good news is that I never had to be the designated driver. But I swear, to this day, that car built character in me like nothing else. I had to hold my head up high and change out my duct tape in the parking lot next to all those Toyota Celicas. That is something that nobody can ever take away.

There were times I was mortified, but there were others where I just threw my hands up in the air and laughed. I believe it was that laughter that helped me hold my head up.

Life isn't going to be perfect all the time, but we have a choice of how we react to the ups and downs. I model this for my kids now, too. When I do or say something stupid, I make sure that they see me laugh it off. I have to teach them that there is a time and a place to be serious, and a time and a place to let ourselves off the hook when we mess up. It feels great to laugh. We should do it as much as we can.

35

W.A.I.T.

> *"Open your mouth only if what you're about to say is more beautiful than silence."*
>
> —ARABIC PROVERB

I told you before that I do and say stupid and embarrassing things all the time. Sometimes I think I should carry around a roll of tape for my mouth! The more I think about it, there are definitely a few people that I am most on edge around and that is when the things come out of my mouth that sound cray-cray. I look around and wonder, who just said that stupid thing? Oh, me! Usually, I can laugh at myself and realize nerve-induced screw-ups are only temporary. Other times I just need to stop where I am and be quiet.

I love the term W.A.I.T. that I learned from one of my teachers, Gabby Bernstein. It stands for:

W - Why
A - Am
I - I
T - Talking

Why am I talking?

As hard as I sometimes hope it'll happen, I am never going to be that shy, quiet girl. I talk, talk, talk, and at times don't even realize what is coming out until it's too late. Lately, I've tried to slow down and be more self-aware of what I'm saying so I don't feel regretful after I talk to people. At times, though, usually when I'm nervous, I will just have word vomit. It's in these times that I ask myself, "Why am I talking?"

If the answer is "I don't know," or "I'm nervous," then I try to just stop. There is absolutely no need to keep an uncomfortable conversation going. One asinine comment doesn't have to lead to more. Instead, I try to change the subject, excuse myself, or bring someone else into the fold to diffuse the situation. There is always a better option than digging the hole deeper until there is no way out.

I have begun to bring more awareness to who makes me nervous and do some deep breathing as they approach me or I am walking up to them to say hello. My goal is to calm my nervous system down before I start talking so I can be less reactive and more responsive. It actually does work!

It is also an option to opt out of a long conversation with someone that you don't feel particularly comfortable around. A polite "hello" is fine. Self-preservation is just as important as making a good impression, so take care of yourself.

Vibes speaker louder than words, meaning not everyone is an energetic match for us. If you don't feel good around someone there is usually a reason—learn to honor that. Always be nice and put your best self forward, but you don't ever have to sacrifice yourself and let your energy plummet around someone.

I have gotten very sensitive to the energy of other people, and I have had to learn to protect myself and clear my energy after I am around a lot of people. I will never forget the day I spent at a holiday bazaar selling t-shirts and signing books for twelve hours. I spoke to hundreds of people, and as the day went on I started to feel totally zapped. By nightfall, I was as weak as could be. I wasn't sure if I caught the flu somehow, that's how bad I felt. I ended up spending the next five days in bed recovering and only getting out to feed my kids, drive them to school, and work with my energy healers. It was a total wake-up call!

I have gotten much smarter about the situations I put myself in, and how I prepare for being around a lot of people. It took five days in bed to figure it out, but it was a lesson I needed to learn.

36

Learn to Forgive Yourself and Others

"When you forgive you don't change the past,
but you do change the future."
—BERNARD MELTZER

This may be the biggest game changer of all. If you take just one thing to better your life from this book, I pray it is from this section.

I am going to get really personal here, even more so than admitting I offered my husband sexual favors for letting me practice meditations on him. My stories are unique to my life, but we all have big bad experiences that were freaking hard, to say the least. Life wouldn't be life without them, yet it is easy to vacillate between wishing they were different and understanding how they helped you grow. I certainly have a list of experiences that are a toss-up. On one hand, I'd love a do-over, but on the other hand they helped me to grow in ways I would never have otherwise. When I think about them like that, the reality is that I know there was a point to them no matter how difficult they made my life, and I could never go back.

We only have one choice, and that is to move forward. These experiences will only hold us back until we make peace with them. They certainly did for me. It took me years to heal and forgive. I can't think of it as wasted time, but I learned a lot about how to forgive, and I will never let anyone or anything hijack my psyche like that again. I am going to share my five steps to true forgiveness with you, but be patient; there are story and background to share first.

Do you remember the very moment that your childhood ended? Like a light switch being turned off—when it turned back on, everything was different. There was no going back.

I remember mine with such vivid detail, and I knew at that moment my life would never be the same.

I wish I had some crazy exciting story for you. Something like how traveling around the world changed me forever, or a sweet memory of how losing my virginity to the love of my life at nineteen made me the woman I am today. That's not the case.

I was called into my principal's office for a secret meeting with my dad, who was on work release while he was serving time in prison. He'd committed a white collar crime, and we were all paying the price right along with him. He told me that his girlfriend didn't want me to live in the house anymore, and since he needed her to take care of the house, I needed to find somewhere to go. Just like that. I was kicked out of my house at fourteen. I asked him what I was supposed to do. Why was my identical twin allowed to stay, but I wasn't? He explained that his girlfriend didn't want me there anymore, he was sorry, and then he gave me a hug and left. And that was that. I had a day or two to figure it out.

I remember walking around my high school campus in a state of shock. I have no idea how I even made it back to class. I asked to go to the bathroom and sat outside on a cold winter day, with the wind blowing through my shirt wondering what the hell I was going to do. I felt like I had been abandoned by the man I loved most in the world, not once but twice: The first time when he was led away from me in handcuffs after being sentenced, and the other was the moment that he chose someone else over me. He chose his girlfriend over his daughter. When I was staring into that cold bleak winter morning, I remember just asking the Universe, "Why?"

By now you are probably wondering where my mother was during all of this. I can't imagine that out of everyone reading this, I am the only product of a horribly messy divorce. My dad announced that he was leaving my mom for another woman. He pretty much left her destitute, brainwashed and manipulated us kids to come with him, and cut off contact with my mom. At this point, I was eleven years old. I didn't speak to my mom for two and a half years and had barely reconciled with her when I got kicked out of the house. Hindsight is 20/20, and, of course, I should have gone directly to live with her no matter how hard I kicked and screamed. But nobody took control of the situation and I ended up living with three different friends over the next several months before finally moving in with my mom.

I was always the kind of kid that pasted a smile on my face no matter what, and that habit followed me into adulthood. I was fourteen, my dad was in jail, I was living with friends, already working five to six days a week, and at any point in time if you asked me how things were going, I would smile and say "Great!" The stress and trauma of what my life was like were just too much for me, and I suppressed everything. Like any teen I just wanted to fit in and be like everyone else.

I convinced myself that I was dealing with so much hardship because I needed a backbone, and I was going to have mounds of character, more than other kids my age, and it would all be worth it.

Time went on and I rebuilt my relationship with my mom and one of my sisters, put myself through college, and landed my dream job in Houston. I was so happy to officially be an adult. I was beyond relieved to be done with the stress of school and worrying if I was making enough in tips to pay my rent. I swear, the day I started my full-time job at Enron you'd think I had hit the lottery, my smile was so big. Remember how much I wanted a Celica? I bought one when I got to Texas, and then promptly realized they are way cooler when you are sixteen.

I had moved halfway across the country to escape my father. I wanted to live somewhere new, so that when someone asked my name I wasn't worried that their first thought would be about my dad. My senior year of college my dad went to prison again, and, honestly, I just needed a fresh start. I worried about my dad all the time, and it was terribly sad for me when he missed my graduation, but I never let my smile fade. I was always "great."

Two years after moving to Houston, I met the man of my dreams and got married. I literally called him my gift from God. I felt that this loving, caring, supportive, and generous man was my reward for dealing with crap for years. You know how people ask, "How did you get so lucky?" Well, you betcha I knew. When Adam was born two years later, everything seemed perfect.

There were moments that would pass as I was rocking my son, thinking about how much I adored him, and I would imagine the anguish that my own mother felt being separated from her children for more than two years. I lovingly took care of every single need for my son, and it would hit me that my mother did this for me.

She loves me just as I love him. What would I do if one day Adam cut me out of his life? How would I survive? How would I face the world? Even though my dad orchestrated situations to manipulate me, I ultimately told my mom that I didn't want to talk to her anymore. The thought of those words coming out of my mouth to the woman that carried me and birthed me, just like I had just done for my children, sent ripples of guilt through me. In the face of such pain, and finally realizing the scope of what I had done, I resorted to my old faithful standby of burying my emotions and moving on.

A little while passed, and my father ran through Philly for the last time and needed a fresh town. He decided to come to Houston. Honestly, there wasn't really anywhere else for him to go. My husband helped to set him up, but here he was, invading the life I had purposefully built away from him. He did what comes naturally, lying and cheating his way through town. I was back on Prilosec from worry, just as I was my senior year of college. My dad threatened suicide every day for weeks, so I lay in bed many nights worrying what the morning would bring. At one point, I painfully told him that he either needed to go ahead and do it already or stop torturing me with his threats. When his money finally ran out again he moved in with us. He lived with us for two years, and then ultimately moved in with my twin sister in New York.

It was painful. I had a love/hate relationship with him. I realized from my experience with my mom that not talking doesn't ever solve the problem. I had one dad, take him or leave him. He was my only option and I couldn't imagine cutting him out of my life. But that didn't mean that I didn't feel triggered by him.

Shortly after my dad moved out, I received the melanoma diagnosis. Fortunately, it was caught very early and was treated with surgery, but it still scared me. I had two young kids and I wanted to be here to raise them.

Within a year of having melanoma I was completely addicted to Ambien and didn't sleep without one for over two years. I had never been a great sleeper, but the thought of going to bed without help got to be so scary that when I tried I would literally sit up the entire night. On top of the Ambien addiction, I was convinced I was going to have a heart attack. I had a ball of anxiety that sat in the middle of my chest 24/7. I would occasionally have heart palpitations as well, and I was convinced that I was going to be one of those young women that had a heart attack and missed every sign. I can't exactly tell you when the ball of anxiety formed in my chest, but I couldn't remember not having it.

For the six months prior to the reading I had with the famous medium, I dabbled here and there in meditation, based on what I read in her books. However, I didn't have a consistent practice until after my reading, when my determination to practice was strengthened as I learned to connect with myself and the world around me through meditation. It felt really natural to me, much more so than I would have thought, and I fell into the rhythm of a daily practice that was consistent and life changing for me.

When I sat in stillness, feelings and emotions that had been suppressed for so many years bubbled to the surface until they spilled out of me. As I became more self-aware I realized that I had to deal with the emotions I had buried. I had pushed them down and pushed them down, but I didn't want to ignore them anymore. I wanted to work through them and get to the other side—and doing so changed my life.

I had days where my meditations ended up with me crying in a ball on the floor. I had never allowed myself to feel, or to process.

The farthest I ever got was telling myself that I was "over" something, which really meant I had made no headway at all.

For about two years, my body and mind were releasing mountains of stress, but when I got to the other side of it all I realized that although it took me twenty-four years to get there, the destination was worth it, and the journey was everything. My journey consisted of five steps, which I now call the Five Steps to True Forgiveness.

The very first step was *awareness*. It's funny, as I was walking my twin sister through these steps, we started laughing. I told her that the very first step took me over twenty years. This wasn't a quick process for me, but it was the most worth-it process that I had ever put myself through.

I could no longer deny the physical and emotional signs that I needed to heal. Some of the physical ones I already mentioned, like the anxiety and the Ambien addiction. I also had mild physical ticks, which started around the time of my parents' divorce. Then there was the melanoma. From the moment I was diagnosed I was convinced that it came from built-up stress in my body. I felt so strongly that I did a little research and found a study linking melanoma to chronic stress. But there were also emotional signs, like being triggered every time I spoke to my dad. Anger and resentment just bubbled to the surface no matter what. Everything annoyed me, and I would just look at him and be completely dragged down by the past.

My mom said something once that always stuck with me, but it took all this time to realize how right she was. She said that living with anger and resentment is like having shackles around you. This makes me think of another quote from Gautama Buddha that says, "Holding onto anger and resentment is like drinking poison and expecting the other person to die."

I knew I had to free myself. I am the only person that had the key to that pair of shackles. The key was forgiveness. I needed to not say I was "over" my dad kicking me out of my house, but I had to forgive him for it with every single cell in my body. I could tell myself all day long that I wasn't responsible for cutting my mom out of my life because I was only eleven, but I had to truly forgive myself for it in order to move on with my life. I was finally ready to be free. I knew that I had to do it myself—not that I had any clue as to what exactly I needed to do, but I decided to go with the flow.

I sat in *stillness* and I let it happen. I let everything swell inside of me until it had no place to go but out of my eyes in the form of tears, and out of my mouth in the form of howls, and out of my hands as they pounded the floor. Stillness some days turned into a storm of emotion that had been buried so deep that it took on a life of its own. I was actually shocked. I didn't know I had it in me. I was proud that I found the courage to dig deep enough to reach those buried places. A few minutes would pass and I would feel calmer, sit back up, get back on my cushion, and be still again. I was so still as I let my body and my subconscious process these emotions and figure out what to do with them. I honestly didn't think. I just sat. I knew something was happening but I couldn't have told you what.

I soon realized it was the RELEASE of all I had held onto for years that dragged me down. After about six weeks of sitting in still-ness every single day without fail, things really started to change. I remember so vividly the day that I was walking my dog and, all of a sudden, it hit me—the ball of anxiety in my chest was gone. Just like that. I don't know at exactly what moment it dissipated, but it was gone so who cares, right?! And it has never come back. That physi-cal shift was a defining moment for me. Imagine carrying around a backpack full of weights all day long, and then one day someone comes and takes it off your back and you feel so light. That is how I felt, just so much lighter. I felt free. I felt so good that I was confident enough to wean off the Ambien. I did extra guided meditations as I fell asleep for a few weeks until I could fall asleep on my own. My ticks didn't completely go away, but they lessened considerably. My body and my mind finally released. They were finally free of the buried emotions that had had a hold on me for so long.

We have all heard the lore of the pot of gold at the end of the rainbow. I found that fortune on the other side of forgiveness when I found *gratitude*.

It became crystal clear to me that part of my purpose in this lifetime was to go through these hardships and to learn how to truly forgive. I didn't get kicked out of the house to prove how strong I was, and I didn't stop talking to my mom to build my character. The purpose of these events was to learn how to truly forgive myself and others. By the end of this process of truly forgiving, I felt gratitude for these experiences. Without them, I would never have this knowledge and the confidence to know that I am capable of finding true forgiveness with every part of me. I came to understand that my Dad was doing the best he could at the time, while wrestling with his own lessons.

Then I realized it was all about *CHOICE*. This last step is kind of like the maintenance step. There are things in life that you obviously cannot control. We can't control what feelings we feel. Our bodies and minds have reactions to things, good and bad. Before we can think, we feel. However, we do have the ability to control what we do with those feelings, or whether we let them control us. Do we allow them to bury themselves deep within us, or do we deal with them as they are happening? Do we sit in stillness and allow our body and mind to process, or do we allow our ego to take over and keep us in a state of perpetual fear?

I chose to exhale the bullshit and inhale the good shit (I didn't make that up, although I wish I had).

You may not have ever noticed before, but after you exhale, before you inhale again, there is a pause. It's brief, but it is there. That is your choice point. What are you going to bring back in? The bullshit or the good shit?

When I make a mistake, I acknowledge the negative feelings about it and exhale them out. I inhale back in the lesson I learned from being part of that situation right along with the peace of seeing how I don't have to let it take me to a dark place. This goes for family, friends, acquaintances, and myself.

Why do I share this story? We all have problems, and we have lived through tough situations. It's possible that you are holding on to some sort of resentment or anger. I am no more special than you. If I can find true forgiveness, so can you. What can you let go of? What are you ready to release? With these five steps of awareness, stillness, release, gratitude, and choice, I am handing you the key to those shackles. Only you can turn it.

37

Get the Money Stuff Under Control

"The quickest way to double your money is to fold it over and put it in your pocket."

—WILL ROGERS

Until I was eleven, my family was the envy of the neighborhood. All people saw were four sweet daughters and a magnificent home. Looking back, I wish I was old enough to appreciate that house, with its sprawling yard and indoor pool. For me, the picture-perfect life is overshadowed with memories of my mom on the phone negotiating payment plans, and at eight years old asking my parents if we had health insurance. Even at a young age, it seemed obvious to me that we were living beyond our means, and I absolutely hated the feeling. I never truly felt secure about money, even before my parent's horrific divorce. After the divorce, there was no denying the fact that we were not in prime financial shape. Our house went up for sheriff's sale and my mom was given absolutely nothing. My dad somehow settled us into another smaller, but still beautiful, home and to this day I am still not sure how bills got paid. I know that many of them didn't, and the creditors driving our cars away in the middle of the night pretty much proved it.

At fourteen I began to take fiscal matters into my own hands and became more responsible for myself. I got a job at a pharmacy because I had a crush on a boy that worked there. I think he only worked there so he could feed his addiction to Carmex, and to this day I cannot see a Carmex container without thinking of my entry into the workforce. I have since decided that there must be some connection between males and medicated lip balm, because my husband uses Carmex too! Nonetheless, it was an easy first job and I had plenty of time to flirt as I stocked the shelves. My boss was kind, and I will never forget the awkward conversation I had with him when I asked him to dock my paycheck in order to pay off my dad's debt to the pharmacy. He graciously patted my hand and told me he appreciated the thought, but I should keep the money I earned. I just couldn't look him in the face unless I offered. I also began babysitting for a customer every Saturday night, and continued that job for four years until I was basically an honorary member of the family. I still keep in touch with them and will never forget their generosity. They went out of their way to find reasons to pay me and supplied me with extra gas money once I could drive.

My crush led to a few dates and then fizzled, mainly because the object of my affection decided he liked my identical twin sister more, which was kind of awkward. I left the pharmacy and moved onto greener pastures in retail for the duration of high school, and then waitressed my way through college.

Most people think of college as the best time in their lives. Those people must have had parents that paid all their bills. College for me

was majorly stressful and I couldn't wait to be done. When I started working, I lived within reasonable means, so paying my bills wasn't a hardship, and I didn't think life could get any better. I shopped sales and discount stores and I knew how to look good on a budget. I paid off my credit card every single month and never let things get out of control. I didn't have a safety net, so there was no way I could let myself get into trouble.

When I got married things got even easier. My husband had worked really hard for ten years and his career was beginning to take off. I could finally stop worrying about finances; I wasn't in it alone anymore, and Mark was incredibly generous.

I never went totally crazy, but I definitely started spending more and enjoying the finer things in life. Mark's favorite line is, "I married a girl that shopped at Loehmann's, and now she wants to shop at Neiman's."

I think that back then I wanted to prove, to myself or to everyone else, that I was finally "normal." My needs began to escalate and I was always thinking about more. I remember when I got my first designer bag from a department store. I visited this Prada bag at Saks for a few months and literally drooled over it. I felt like if I could just have that bag, I wouldn't need another. I would be so happy with that black bag and it would go with everything. On probably my fourth or fifth "visit" I bought the bag. It was a really big deal, as I had never spent that much on one item before. I wore that bag proudly, and I still have it today. It is beautiful and I have taken amazing care of it; almost ten years later it looks like new.

But a few months after that purchase my desire for more grew. All of a sudden, I needed a brown bag, and cool shoes, and then I needed Lululemon tank tops in every color. I was never complete. I actually kept a list in my phone of everything I "needed." I was always on the hunt for more, and then when I got it there was always something else.

When I think about that list I cringe, but it was all part of my journey. What makes me the saddest, though, is how I thought that my worth was tied in some way to purses and Gucci belts. I truly felt that I needed these things to be whole and feel proud of myself.

After a few years, I was starting to make myself sick. I didn't want to constantly be on the hunt for more, and I wanted to learn to be happy with or without fancy things. As I became more self-aware and began transforming my life, the reality of my money baggage became even more obvious, and I felt ready to make a change.

I acknowledged that I had blocks related to money but I wasn't ready to face them until recently when I began to feel that they were holding me back in my life. I took an online course about money and it finally opened my eyes to what was holding me back (if you have money stuff to deal with, check out amandafrances.com, and tell her I sent you!). It forced me to face the fears and baggage that I carried with me regarding finances. I came to realize that the reason I felt the need to buy so much, and many times multiples of things, was because I was scared that one day I wouldn't be able to. What if our money disappeared and I couldn't shop anymore? I had a deep-rooted need to buy everything I could now in case I couldn't have it later. This led me to overspending and buying multiples of things "just in case." The thought of running out of something totally freaked me out. If my shampoo was halfway finished I needed a new one. If I liked a shirt in black, then I had to buy the gray and white too, just in case. This behavior never got so out of control that it caused a problem in my marriage or bank account, but it made me feel desperate and materialistic.

Finally admitting that this pattern was an issue and acknowledging my lack mentality was a game-changer for me. Using positive affirmations and learning to respect my money by actually keeping track of what I spent made a huge difference. I stopped feeding into that lack mentality, and began to feel secure and abundant. I vividly remember one night that was a real turning point for me. I was at the drugstore buying cuticle cream, and, ordinarily, I would have bought three—one to keep at my desk, one in my purse, and one for the car, just in case I ran out in another location. I had three in my hand and I paused, silently repeated an affirmation, and then put two away. I looked at the shelf and saw that there was an entire row of cream. It would be there when I needed more, and I would be able to afford it then as well. I had tears in my eyes as I checked out with ONE cream. That was truly a milestone for me.

As I stopped overspending I began to feel more abundant in every way. I realized I had enough—enough food in the pantry, enough makeup, enough to wear, and enough books on my Kindle. I didn't need to download every title at once. God willing, when I truly needed something, I would be able to have it.

I started saying a mantra about money, and I kept it on an index card in my wallet and in my car. I would read it and say it aloud before I went into stores. It went like this:

"I have enough. I am enough. I am safe. My life is stable. Money will not disappear before my eyes. I consistently have enough money for my needs and desires, therefore I do not need to satisfy them all at once."

If I could talk to myself ten years ago, I would implore a younger Ali not to get caught up in feeling that "things" defined her. I would convince her to get to know herself and be honest about what really makes her happy. I'd tell her to learn to be satisfied, and don't ever make it about keeping up with anyone else. She has nothing to prove except how beautiful her soul is. It is okay to enjoy nice things, and she should, but they don't define her in any way. Material things come and go, so put her full attention on loving and caring for those around her, serving the world, and on finding out who the person is behind her eyes.

It's funny. Now that "things" do not define me, I enjoy what I have much more, and I crave much less. These days I'd rather have energy healing sessions over a new purse any day!

38

Be Honest About the Time Things Take

"Once she stopped rushing through life, she was amazed how much more life she had time for."

—UNKNOWN

I used to tell myself that I could get anywhere in town in about five minutes. I would race around trying to squeeze in just one more errand, and I was always stressed. I was unrealistic about the time things took. Errands, phone calls, making dinner—all of these things took way more time than I was allotting for them.

Once I began slowing down in other areas of my life, I realized I needed to have a better game plan for how I was handling the everyday tasks in my life. Part of that was being realistic about the time needed to accomplish certain tasks. I always felt just short of what I needed in terms of time, and I can see now that it was another way that I was living with a lack mentality. I always felt that my day would have been better if I just had another twenty minutes to get one more thing done. I always felt one step behind, and who wants to go through life like that?

I got honest with myself and shifted my mentality regarding time from one of lack to one of abundance. Once I felt that time was on my side, much of the stress regarding errands and to-dos melted away. I no longer tried to squeeze too many things into a short time frame, but I began to plan out what needed to be done and chose only what could fit into the time I had.

I would never go so far as to say that I love running errands now, but I don't mind them because they don't stress me out like they used to. Of course, I'd rather be meditating, on a run, sipping tea with a friend, or writing, but caring for myself and a family does make errands a necessity. I went from dreading errands to feeling neutral about them.

Sometimes I spread them out, and do one a day, but usually I save them up and take a few hours one afternoon to get everything knocked out.

I learned a trick from Judy, my spiritual life counselor, which changed my life. She taught me how to expand time.

The old me would be a nut case if I got held up and couldn't cross everything off my list that I hoped to accomplish in an allotted time. I could plan all I wanted, but things like traffic, getting stuck behind a train, and long lines slowed things down, and I had no control over them. I remember how my heart would race, and I would feel panicked because carpool time was quickly approaching and I wasn't through with my list. But now, I simply expand time.

I take a deep breath and relax my body, and in a calm and sure way I say with intention, "I expand time." I don't just say it a few times, but I truly feel from the bottom of my heart that it is true and time will expand for me. Then I surrender, let go, and allow the Universe to work its magic.

Every time I use this trick, something happens that works out in my favor. In fact, the very first time I used it I was amazed at the result.

We were on our way to my son's baseball lesson and we were stuck in major traffic. These lessons are not cheap, and since we basically pay by the minute I really wanted to get there on time, but it was pretty obvious that was not going to happen. I was doing some deep breathing while we were at a standstill on the freeway and I remembered the expanding time trick that Judy had taught me a few hours earlier. I decided to try it because at this point I had nothing to lose. I said, "I expand time" with intention a few times and then simply let go emotionally. The minutes were ticking away, and we pulled up to the lesson twenty-five minutes late, but at least I was still calm, cool, and collected. My son would just use the last five minutes, and there was nothing much I could do.

We walked in and I immediately apologized to his teacher and explained that I understood we would only have five minutes. He replied, "Don't worry, the person after you canceled, so you can still have a full lesson."

A huge smile crossed my lips, and I knew in my heart that because I stayed calm and expanded time, it had all worked out.

I still have days where the thought crosses my mind that it would be nice to have one more hour in the day. Some of this comes from the fact that my kids stay up later now and I don't have two or three hours after they go to bed to myself anymore. If I am sticking to my 10:30 p.m. bedtime I may have an hour at best. The difference is my attitude about it. I have tasks that are time-sensitive that I prioritize, and I have others that simply get moved to the next day or week on my calendar. I want to accomplish them, but the world won't fall apart if it takes a few more days. I decided that I can stress or I can deal, and there is no way I am going back to that stress.

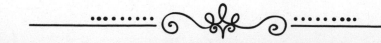

39

Learn to Veg

"Take time to do what makes your soul happy."
—UNKNOWN

I really thought for years that in order to be productive I had to be on the go every minute of the day. There were days that I never even sat down. I did everything from prepping meals to doing dishes, to straightening up, to exercising, walking the dogs, playing with the kids, errands, plans, and who knows what else. Once I started working and teaching, those things still needed to be done, but on top of that I had to plan for classes and actually teach them. I would try to read or enjoy a show when I got into bed, but by then I was so exhausted I could hardly keep my eyes open.

Learning to slow down was not easy for me. By now you know that I consider meditation to be the biggest tool for transformation that I have, and it has touched so many areas of my life, including this one. When I am sitting in stillness there is nothing as important as simply being in the moment. Everything else can wait. My kids know not to disturb me unless someone throws up, is bleeding, or they think we need to call 911. All of my responsibilities and to-dos melt away for those precious minutes.

It was pretty eye-opening to see that when I take twenty to thirty minutes and step away from it all, nothing falls apart.

Every so often now I simply veg out. I let my kids have a bit of downtime every day after school before they start homework or we run off to an activity. There are many days that I am preparing dinner, washing lunch kits, and signing tests, but I have started to relax with them a bit. If they are reading on the couch I grab my book and join them. If they are watching a show I may watch one on my iPad next to them. I realize that they just want to be near me, and I just want to be near them, so I can't even tell you who loves the closeness more. There have been so many times that my kids have asked me to come sit with them on the couch and I have given reasons why I can't. I don't want them to remember me only saying, "I can't because I have to get X, Y, or Z done." I want them to remember that sometimes I said "Yup!" and laid down next to them and snuggled. Every once in a while, it feels amazing to take a break and just veg.

40

What Do You Stand For?

"The things you are passionate about are not random. They are your calling."

—FAVIENNE FREDRICKSON

One of my final and favorite assignments during my meditation teacher certification program was to think about my guiding principles and develop a personal credo.

So often as moms, our identity is tied into our family and responsibilities, but this was an opportunity to really think about who I am as a person, and what is important to my soul going forward in my life.

My personal credo is Faith, Compassion, Light.

Have Faith—I have faith that every experience serves a purpose in my life. With a little distance, I can see clearly that each and every experience in my past shaped me and allowed me to grow and become more in touch with my spirituality. This isn't just about the past, however. I have faith that my life will unfold just as it is supposed to.

When I am unsure which path I should follow, I have faith that I am not alone on this journey. I know that I will be divinely guided to the right opportunities, relationships, and situations that will allow me to reach my full potential in this lifetime. This faith leads me to compassion.

Be Compassionate—I strongly believe that we need to show compassion to everyone on this earth, including ourselves. When we truly love and accept ourselves we can give more fully to those around us. Judging others serves no one; instead, we need to foster acceptance knowing that nobody is perfect, including ourselves. Forgiving ourselves can set us free, and forgiving one another sets us free as well. We forgive through compassion, with the faith that we can choose a better, more peaceful way to live.

We all make mistakes, and when they occur it is our job to learn the lessons from them and use the experiences as stepping stones to personal growth. The mistakes don't define us, what we learn from them does. This compassion for ourselves and others leads to light.

Share My Light—When we truly love and accept ourselves we can share all that is good in us, or our light, with the world. It is an honor, privilege, and responsibility to bring this gift to the world. Sharing our light with others allows us to connect in a deep and profound way. In order to do this with true authenticity we must be vulnerable at times, but with faith and compassion, we can confidently aim to make the world a better place.

What you give you also attract, so it is imperative to give your best to the world each and every day, and to approach every situation from a place of love and kindness. If we strive to share our light and to be the best version of ourselves every day, the universe will reward us with an abundance of love and light in return.